JOURNAL
of
WONDER

366 days of musical inspiration to reflect upon
and soothe your soul

CLEMENCY BURTON-HILL

First published in 2023 by Headline Home
an imprint of Headline Publishing Group

The majority of the text in this volume was originally published in
Year of Wonder (9781472251824) and *Another Year of Wonder* (9781472259370).
Published in 2017 and 2021 by Headline Home.

1

All chapter openers: manuscript score of the violoncello part of the B-Minor Mass by
J. S. Bach. Dresden, *Sächsische* Landesbibliothek – Staats und Universitätsbibliothek,
D-Dl Mus.2405-D-21. Photo: Alfredo Dagli Orti/REX/Shutterstock.

Cataloguing in Publication Data is available from the British Library

ISBN 978 1035 41214 3
e-ISBN 978 1035 41215 0

Typeset by EM&EN
Printed and bound in Great Britain by Clays Ltd, Elcograf S.p.A.

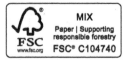

HEADLINE PUBLISHING GROUP
An Hachette UK Company
Carmelite House
50 Victoria Embankment
London EC4Y 0DZ

www.headline.co.uk
www.hachette.co.uk

Contents

Introduction

Journalling is an age-old human practice, as is making – and listening to – classical music. Both writing and music can be a powerful and accessible route to personal insight, emotional clarity and transformation – to say nothing of being a shortcut to joy, beauty and wonder. And, as many psychological and neuroscientific studies have shown, something magical happens when we do both of these things together. We know that the human brain has a unique neural circuitry that is activated; a circuitry that could lead to heightened creativity, even the possibility of healing. In our ever-more-perplexing world, where the promise of both creativity and healing are peddled to us almost constantly – but not always in the most sustainable of ways – I hope this little listening and writing project can restore some creative equilibrium, some reinvigoration, some hope, in your life. All you really need for this journal is a way to listen to the music that is contained in these pages – all of which is available on the internet (although I urge you to listen, if you are able, via one of the many services available that offer compensation for the artists!) – and an ability to listen, *internally*. In other words: a little bit of time; a little bit of curiosity about yourself and your fellow human beings over the centuries; a little technological assistance, but most importantly: open ears and a very open heart.

I am not going to assume that you have an ability to journal long-hand – since my brain unexpectedly ruptured in 2020, I have not been able to do that myself – but, if you have the ability to write your entries using a pen and paper, I hope you can. If not – no matter. The main thing is that you are here, showing up for yourself in all of your questioning, all of your wondering, all of your listening. And that is a beautiful thing. A journal – whether physical or digital – can help us work out certain life niggles and obstacles, whether large or small. It can help with overwhelming questions personal and professional, local and global, all within a private container. It can expand, pretty much infinitely, to be an unlimited space for safely confronting self-doubts, uncertainties, frustrations and other uncomfortable feelings that are inevitably part of being human. And, the best part of all, by a mystical process of emotional and neurological alchemy, that act of bravery – of actually confronting the reality that you are facing – often leads to processing, even accepting, that reality. Not immediately, obviously, and not necessarily fully. But it's a terrific start.

A word about dates. Sometimes, I have tied a particular entry to a particular date. Sometimes I have not. I hope your own *Journal of Wonder* entries will give you a helpful chronological framework to reflect back upon, when the year is over, but if for some reason the musical entry doesn't yield nourishing insights for you on that particular date, again: no matter. There are plenty more of them; please don't force anything. I hope you will use this journal – and its music – whichever way you feel most supported; to help you access your individual observations, feelings, emotions, ideas, cycles, patterns, rhythms. Even if the music itself on a particular day is not acoustically calming or soothing, per se, being able to cultivate an awareness of your personal response – having the key to *access* yourself – should be very focusing, and a source of deep inspiration, motivation and, yes, serenity.

Like any new habit, though, it might not be easy at first. I recommend managing expectations and starting small. Go easy on yourself, be patient, but also try to be consistent. Many of these musical pieces are just a few minutes long. Use the prompts, along with the music, as you will. Jot. Bullet. List. No one is expecting complete sentences; in fact no one is expecting anything! This is for you. Maybe start with stream of consciousness, or note down something you already know or can easily remember. (And I don't

mean any 'facts' about classical music, by the way! This is not a test,
I repeat, this is not a test.)

Today I'm thinking about . . .
Today I am remembering . . .
Today I am feeling . . .
Today I am wondering . . .
Today I am hoping for . . .
Three things I am grateful for . . .
Three things I could let go of . . .
Even: three things I want off my to-do list . . .

Ask yourself some questions.

How do I feel when I listen to this?
What comes up for me?
Where does that feel in my body?
Did it stay there?
What do I think I need?
What do I think others could need from me?
How could I possibly build steps to make that happen?
What's my next realistic step?

Use these open questions, accompanied by the music, to take
yourself deeper within yourself. How easy is it for you to access
the most reflective or more emotional part of yourself? If you are
hearing a narrative in the music, what do you think that is reflecting?
   A diary offers you a safe place to record your feelings and work
through your emotions. I believe the same thing could be said of
music too. In fact, I know it is all these things – and so much more
besides.
   I guarantee that whatever is going on in your heart and soul, all
of the composers included in this book have experienced something
akin to that and will have created a piece of very precise music so

it connects directly with you. There is no map, or key, or code to decode while listening to the pieces. If something resonates in you and it can help you with your mental state, it is the beauty of this 'double journal'. The composers all needed to write this music to express what was in their brains, just like you can unleash your thoughts by writing in a journal.

May you find joy in these pages.
May you find peace, too.
May you find comfort.
And clarity.
And if not: there is always tomorrow.

Thank you for being here.

Clemency Burton-Hill

November 2023

Welcome. We are just at the start of this musical journey together.
Take a moment to reflect on any particular aspect of the past year,
or on all of it. What are you thankful for? What are your hopes
for the year to come?

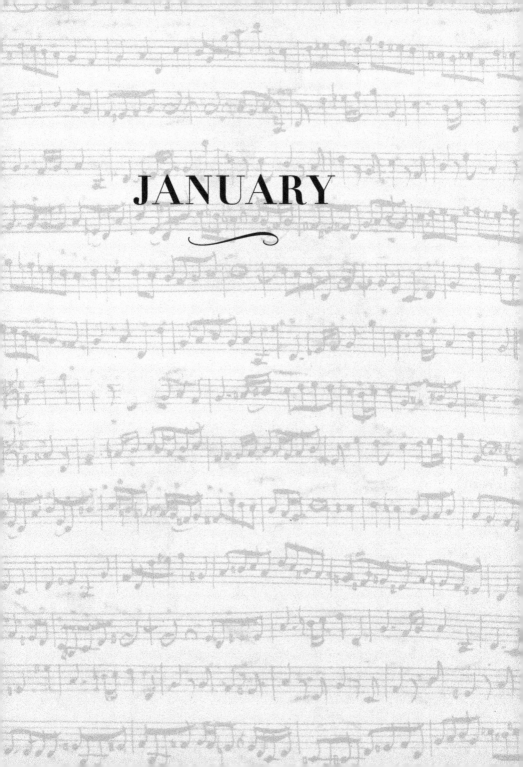

JANUARY

Jesu, nun sei gepreiset – Jesus, now be praised
Cantata BWV 41
1: Chorus
by Johann Sebastian Bach (1685–1750)

1

And we're off! What a thing it is, to embark on an entire new journey around the sun. But who to choose as our musical companion on day one? It has to be Johann Sebastian Bach and this rousing chorus from a New Year's Day cantata. Whoever you are, and wherever you are, I sincerely hope this lifts your spirits on the first day of January. We have a big year ahead of us: let us link arms on this adventure together; let us go!

Étude **in C major, op. 10 no. 1**
by Frédéric Chopin (1810–1849)

2

It can be a funny old day, 2 January, and sometimes a bit anticlimactic, but this two-minute piece seems to me to encapsulate all the promise of the new year – with its attendant hopes and dreams, discoveries, resolutions and potential revolutions . . .

3

O virtus sapientiae
by Hildegard of Bingen (c. 1098–1179)

Hildegard of Bingen was a nun, a writer, a scientist, a philosopher, a prophet and a Christian visionary. Somehow, this remarkable human also found the time to compose at least seventy pieces of music, most with their own original poetic texts. This would be vibrant and unusual music if it were written in any era; that it was written almost a thousand years ago, by a very busy nun, only heightens the wonder.

4

Asteroid 4179: Toutatis
by Kaija Saariaho (b. 1952)

Celestial bodies have long held a deep fascination for composers. Finnish composer Kaija Saariaho here focuses her terrific musical imagination on an asteroid. Specifically, the stony asteroid whose orbit passes closest to Earth. I love the idea of this plucky, individualistic asteroid, our closest neighbour, doing its own thing, crisscrossing the sky in its own special time and colliding with other heavenly objects in its own, unrepeatable way.

Try to listen to one piece a day and use the music as a prompt for your journalling. Notice which pieces you prefer. There are no rules here, I promise, but as the year unfolds, try to note which ones seem to help release something in you.

5

Crucifixus
by Antonio Lotti (c. 1667–1740)

I find this music radiant, moving, magnificent. If you can take three and a half minutes to stop whatever you're doing and just let it wash over you, do it.

6

Cello Suite no. 1 in G major
1: Prelude
by Johann Sebastian Bach (1685–1750)

Each of Bach's six cello suites has its own distinct personality, its own story, its own blend of heart-stopping beauty and high-jinks joy. I could have chosen any movement, but I have started at the very beginning, with the opening movement of the opening suite, in the ardent hope that at some point, maybe now, maybe later, you'll find the time to go on and listen to them all – to take them into your life and let them enrich your every day.

Sonata for cello and piano
2: 'Cavatine'
by Francis Poulenc (1899–1963)

7

Poulenc, who died on this day, led a complex, colourful life: he was openly gay, was possibly active in the French resistance, and the early levity and lightheartedness you can hear in his earlier music was later tempered by a gravity produced perhaps by the difficult experiences life had thrown his way. He began sketching out this richly sensuous cello sonata in 1940; i.e. in the shadow of World War Two. I think it's beautiful.

again (after ecclesiastes)
by David Lang (b. 1957)

8

Happy birthday to one of contemporary music's greats: the Pulitzer-winning composer David Lang. His is a music of fierce humanity and, for all its cerebral intelligence, he peddles in immediate emotional connection. *'If you use these pieces to figure out who you are and what you believe,'* he says, *'you can dedicate a huge amount of energy to really trying to figure out what's true.'*

9

Sonata in F Minor for two pianos, op. 34b
2: Andante, un poco adagio
by Johannes Brahms (1833–1897)

In the Romantic era, it was indubitably Johannes Brahms who contributed most significantly to the genre. This piece actually began life as a string quintet, and was subsequently rearranged as a popular piano quintet, but it's this version, for two pianos, that really does it for me.

10

Violin Sonata no. 2
1. Allegro non troppo
by Germaine Tailleferre (1892–1983)

Today, we have a fresh and lovely violin sonata from one of the coolest cats of twentieth-century music. As the only female member of the avant-garde Parisian group Les Six, she met the prevailing prejudice against women composers head on, by all accounts simply refusing to let it stop her. I love the fact that she was apparently still to be found composing at her piano right up to the day she died, in her early nineties.

What draws you to classical music and why? Is it to relax and unwind? Is it to help you concentrate? Is it to help you get unstuck or to give you a different energy? Music, while just 'sonorous air', is powerful: consider how you could harness it to help you get more of the things you need or want.

11

Ave, dulcissima Maria
by Morten Lauridsen (b. 1943)

As our Western societies become ever more secular, there is a real and growing hunger for spiritually inflected music that seems to fill a void or meet a real human need. And so – whoever you are, whatever you're up to – I hope you can find eight or so minutes to carve out the space to simply let this into your life today. I promise you'll thank yourself for it.

12

Octet in E flat major, op. 20
1. Allegro moderato ma con fuoco
by Felix Mendelssohn (1809–1847)

As birthday presents go, this has to be one of the all-time greats.

Felix Mendelssohn wrote this exuberant piece of chamber music as a birthday gift for his great friend and violin teacher, Edward Rietz. He was sixteen years old. '*I had a most wonderful time in the writing of it*,' he later admitted – and what I particularly love is that you can hear that enjoyment in every note.

Deux arabesques, L. 66
1: Andantino con moto in E major
by Claude Debussy (1862–1918)

This supremely graceful vignette is about four minutes long, a snap, yet has the ability to instantly slow down my world; to drench everything in light. And if that's not a precious quality for a cold winter day, I don't know what is.

Reverie
by Angela Morley (1924–2009)

With two Emmy awards under her belt, Angela Morley made history when she became the first openly transgender person to be nominated for an Oscar, in 1974. (She was nominated again in 1976.) It's easy to overuse the word pioneer, but I feel like we should just let that fact rest there for a moment. She died on this day in 2009.

15

Quatuor pour la fin du temps – Quartet for the End of Time
5: *Louange à l'éternité de Jesus*
by Olivier Messiaen (1908–1992)

Here's another example of music as a form of spiritual resistance so moving it stops me in my tracks. When France fell in 1940 Messiaen was rounded up and deported to a German camp. Among his fellow prisoners in Stalag VIII-A were a clarinettist, a violinist and a cellist. Messiaen managed to procure some paper and a small pencil and in circumstances it's impossible to comprehend, put together the work that many consider to be his masterpiece.

16

20 Exercices et Préludes
1: Vivace
by Maria Szymanowska (1789–1831)

I find this fizzy little prelude a perfect pick-me-up: a quick musical fix that instantly gets me in the mood to get things done.

Adelita
by Francisco Tarrega (1852–1909)

17

Look, sometimes what I really need in life is an epic symphony with all the bells and whistles, and sometimes what I need is a tiny little shot of musical perfection. Lyrical, bittersweet, touching, this miniature by one of the founding fathers of the classical guitar does what it does in under two minutes and is all the more delicious for it.

Habanera
by Emmanuel Chabrier (1841–1894)

18

Emmanuel Chabrier, who was born on this day, was discouraged by his bourgeois family from following his heart into music. He dutifully studied law and worked as a civil servant in the French Ministry of the Interior for many years, composing as much as he could in his spare time, until, on the cusp of turning forty, he decided (and I paraphrase) that life's too short. Once he decided to take the plunge, he wrote often-effervescent music that seems almost drunk on life, and remained a full-time composer for the rest of his days.

Focus on the feelings you want to embrace for the year ahead.
Would you like more joy, more gratitude, more satisfaction?
Where, and with whom? Reflect on some ways you could
bring this into your life.

Electric Counterpoint
1: Fast
by Steve Reich (b. 1936)

19

In this hypnotic piece for electric guitar virtuoso and tape, Reich constantly teases our expectations about tune and accompaniment in a way that would have been familiar to composers of, say, the eighteenth century. And when it comes to those mesmerizing patterns that develop and build in our ear, he's walking a direct line from J. S. Bach. Consider this a supreme January mood-booster . . .

On the Nature of Daylight
by Max Richter (b. 1966)

20

Like the very greatest works of art, this gut-wrenchingly beautiful track contains multitudes: beauty and grief, love and loss, interiority and presence; everything.

21

Berceuse
by Amy Beach (1867–1944)

Today's spotlight shines a light on another pioneer – a woman who refused to let the casual but total bias against her gender stop her. A prodigious talent and virtuoso pianist, Amy Beach was essentially forbidden by her husband from performing in public or publishing her work. But that did not stop her from writing reams of music, of which this gorgeous lullaby is a particularly luscious example.

22

Piano Sonata
2: Lent
by Henri Dutilleux (1916–2013)

I want to get on the meditation bandwagon. I really do. But the truth is: I struggle. Enter music. To me, this piece is like a secret free hack to get me in the same headspace, if I really open up my ears and allow it to do its work. The net effect is similar, and it costs nothing. Incredible.

Sure on this shining night
by Samuel Barber (1910–1981)

23

To a titan of American arts today, who died on this day. Samuel Barber was a professional baritone, a highly respected conductor, and, most importantly, an iconic composer, much lauded even in his own lifetime. He had an innate gift for direct and emotive melody. And yet he struggled with depression and alcoholism, and his creative life was dogged by many periods of writer's block.

Mass for Five Voices
5: Agnus Dei
by William Byrd (c. 1539/40–1623)

24

I love how the writing here is supremely controlled yet somehow sensual in its clarity. Listen how, for example, with each successive invocation of the Agnus Dei, he seamlessly folds in a new vocal line, as though we are listening in on a private conversation which eventually unspools to a magnificent, moving climax involving all the voices.

25

Scottish Fantasy, op. 46
4: Finale (Allegro guerriero)
by Max Bruch (1838–1920)

For Burns Night, music from a German composer who had no obvious personal connection to bonnie Scotland but was so taken by the richness and vibrancy of its folk music tradition that he wrote an entire fantasia based on some of its best tunes. I hope Bruch's music gets your feet tapping and perhaps has you marvelling anew at ways in which music can connect us across space, geography and time.

26

Unsent Love Letters
by Elena Kats-Chernin (b. 1957)

Inspired by the unsent love letters of avant-garde French composer Erik Satie, Elena Kats-Chernin has written a suite of twenty-six exquisite piano miniatures, each one reflecting some element of Satie's wholly unique art, love and life. If you can listen with a classic French drink in hand, so much the better . . .

Symphony no. 41 in C major, K. 551 ('Jupiter')
4: Molto allegro
by Wolfgang Amadeus Mozart (1756–1791)

27

It's a clichéd word, genius, and so hard to quantify, but I think we can all agree that this guy was the real deal: a child prodigy, probably the most gifted writer of melody there has ever been or will ever be, a composer of music so profound, so wise, so witty and tender and empathetic and human that its being in the world simply makes things a little bit better.

'What power art thou' ('Cold Song')
from *King Arthur*
by Henry Purcell (1659–1695)

28

Sometimes the greatest power comes from simplicity. Purcell pretty much builds this piece around a single note, ramping up tension through the repeated bassline (his trademark) and driving John Dryden's words hypnotically forward through evocative frosted strings and shimmering, chromatic harmony. It's an immediately arresting, weird and unforgettable work, a fitting example of the sort of brilliance which made Purcell one of the most significant musicians the UK has ever produced.

We are one month in! Do any of the pieces particularly stand out for you? Check in on 31 December and notice how/if the music has changed you, even a little bit . . .

'Time Lapse' – piano version
by Michael Nyman (b. 1944)

29

This was originally written for the 1985 film *A Zed & Two Noughts*, and remarkably, director Peter Greenaway actually asked for the music to be written and recorded *before* he started shooting. This haunting track is a stunningly beautiful work, whose solemn power derives from Nyman's superb use of what's known in music as 'ground bass', a repeating 'ostinato' chord sequence that becomes, essentially, the music's pulse, its beating heart.

Lowak Shoppala' – Fire and Light
Act I: VIII: 'Koni'
by Jerod Impichchaachaaha' Tate (b. 1968)

30

The distinguished composer Jerod Impichchaachaaha' Tate is a citizen of the Chickasaw Nation, the thirteenth-largest federally recognized Native Peoples group in the US. Today's piece is from a visionary work expressing Chickasaw culture, history and identity through modern classical music, children's voices, art and drama, which Tate created with three other Chickasaw artists. I find this very moving.

31

Four Impromptus, op. 90 D. 899
No. 3 in G flat
by Franz Schubert (1797–1828)

Let us mark the close of this first month of the year with a piece that celebrates a major musical birthday. Franz Schubert, born on this very day, is one of the heroes of the Romantic era: in his tragically short life (he died at thirty-one), he pretty much single-handedly established the German art song ('lieder') tradition, writing more than six hundred of them, many of which remain shining masterpieces of the form; he also composed symphonies, piano sonatas, song cycles, masses, operas and dozens of miniatures such as today's short piano work.

The 'impromptu' was all the rage in nineteenth-century musical circles, and Schubert deftly turned his hand to the form, spinning an entire narrative world in just a few minutes. I struggled to choose which impromptu to select for today, but honestly they're so short, and so very sweet, you could do far worse than to enjoy the whole lot.

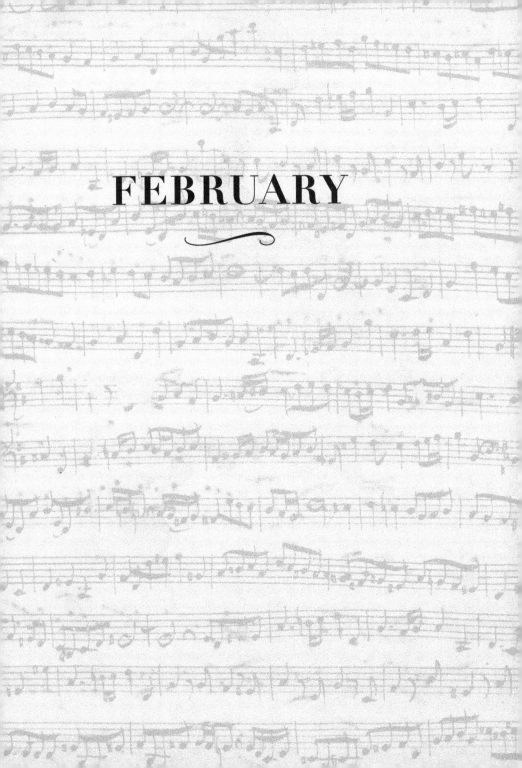

FEBRUARY

Oboe Concerto in D minor, op. 1
2: Adagio
by Alessandro Ignazio Marcello (1673–1747)

1

For my money, this is quite simply one of the most beautiful pieces ever written for one of the most beautiful instruments out there. Mournful, yet somehow hovering on the edges of an exquisite hopefulness at the same time, I find it all the more moving when I listen to it today, the day Marcello died. I'll say no more and let the music speak for itself.

Alma redemptoris mater
by Giovanni Pierluigi da Palestrina (1525–1594)

2

Today we'll hear one of Palestrina's motets, his setting of a Marian hymn praising 'the Mother of our Saviour'. I am often amazed by how something that sounds so ethereal and otherworldly can connect us to something so fundamentally human. Again and again, I marvel at this irrefutable fact: that human beings come together, and sing. In dark times, in all times, I find it offers such simple but profound consolation.

3

'Il cavalier di Spagna' – 'A Spanish Knight'
from *La liberazione di Ruggiero dall'isola d'Ancina*
by Francesca Caccini (c. 1587–1641)

It was on this day in Florence in 1625 that the work generally regarded as the first opera ever composed by a woman was given its premiere. Francesca Caccini was a talented singer, lutenist, poet and teacher. As a member of the court of the Grand Duchess of Tuscany, Maria Maddalena, she would almost certainly have been considered one of the most influential female European composers of her time. Sadly, very little of her music survives.

4

Schlaflied
by Sven Helbig (b. 1968)

As well as being a gifted composer, the German musician Sven Helbig is also a director, instrumentalist, arranger and producer, as fluent in electronics and other digital technologies as he is in traditional counterpoint and harmony. He co-founded the Dresden Symphony Orchestra specifically with a mission to perform only contemporary music, and his dynamic versatility across multiple platforms has led him to create some of the most interesting work of our time.

12 Fantasias for flute without bass
1: Fantasia in A major
by Georg Philipp Telemann (1681–1767)

5

Cast your mind, if you will, way back in time to the depths of the Ice Age. While some homo sapiens were busy carving figurative sculptures, others of the species were apparently filling their caves with the sound of music produced by bone and ivory flutes. The thought of these early people gives me actual shivers: something to ponder, perhaps, as you listen to Telemann's swirling, freewheeling virtuosics. Aren't humans amazing?

Elégie in C minor, op. 24
by Gabriel Fauré (1845–1924)

6

'A direct expression of pathos' is how one of Fauré's biographers describes this unashamedly lush yet quietly intimate work. As a composer, Fauré bridges an interesting moment in musical history, with pieces such as this one exemplifying a sort of high French Romanticism which would soon give way to the cooler stance and more intellectual approach of avant-garde modernism.

Do you have any pre-conceived views of classical music? Note them here and come back to them as you journey through the book. Are you hoping to build a new relationship with it? In what way(s)?

Miserere
by Gregorio Allegri (c. 1582–1652)

7

Allegri, who died on this day, composed the now iconic *Miserere* for the Tenebrae service in Holy Week which began at dusk. During the service, all the candles in the chapel would have been slowly extinguished, one by one, until finally there was a lone candle burning – which was then hidden. It must have been incredibly atmospheric.

Piano Trio
1: 'Pale Yellow'
by Jennifer Higdon (b. 1962)

8

The American composer Jennifer Higdon says she has always been fascinated with the connection between painting, colours and music, often picturing colours as she composes. For me this meditative piano trio in all its pale yellow glory conveys a mood of absolute reflection, and thus delivers me into a sort of state of grace.

9

'For Jóhann'
by Vikingur Ólafsson (b. 1984)

On this day in 2018 the contemporary music world lost one of its most distinctive voices, the Icelandic composer Jóhann Gunnar Jóhannsson. This touching tribute from his countryman, the brilliant young pianist Vikingur Ólafsson, takes music by J. S. Bach as its principal inspiration but pays subtle homage to Jóhannsson's own style. I find it to be intensely moving: three short minutes that, with so little, do so much.

10

Agnus Dei
by Charlotte Bray (b. 1982)

First performed on this day in 2016, this setting of the Agnus Dei is a compelling example of how classical music exists in dialogue across the centuries. Bray was directly inspired by William Byrd's five-part Mass, and in particular the Agnus Dei movement. Like Byrd, Bray at first uses just three voices of the ensemble, layering them until finally all five parts of the ensemble are heard together in a powerful, uplifting climax.

Nunc dimittis
by Arvo Pärt (b. 1935)

11

To a piece of sacred choral music today that was composed this century but feels somehow eternal, as if suspended in space and time. If you can spare around seven minutes of your day to close your eyes, hit pause on everything else and let this piece in, truly in, I'm quite sure you won't regret it.

6 Consolations
No. 3 in D flat major
by Franz Liszt (1811–1886)

12

It is mid-February. Be consoled by this – just this.

13

The Currents
by Sarah Kirkland Snider (b. 1973)

I love Sarah Kirkland Snider's emphasis on storytelling and narrative; it's a reminder of one of the great gifts of music: you can listen, let your mind wander, and map your own story onto whatever you hear. There are no rules.

14

Étude no. 2
by Philip Glass (b. 1937)

I don't wish to dwell upon the fact that today is Valentine's Day – a needlessly difficult day for many – but I hope you will forgive me a little indulgence, in the form of a short musical love-gift to myself. An act of 'self-care', if you will.

Because: my adoration for this piece knows no bounds. See you tomorrow.

Many of these composers had to make serious sacrifices for their art. Many didn't achieve success or gain recognition in their lifetimes. Think about any goals you might have. What can you put in place to help you achieve them? What would success look like for you?

15

Fandango
by Santiago de Murcia (1673–1739)

Creatively way ahead of its time, de Murcia's music has a rhythmic effervescence that reliably gets my feet tapping. And yet, despite his vision and inventiveness, he died a pauper. Stories like his come up again and again in the history of music: these towering creative minds, ignored in their day, who could never have imagined how their music might live on and light up future lives. Something to think about as you press play.

16

Piano Quartet in E flat major, op. 47
3: Andante cantabile
by Robert Schumann (1810–1856)

Robert Schumann – who suffered from devastating bouts of depression, who tried to take his own life, who ended his days in an asylum and was dead by forty-six – is an intensely autobiographical composer. Here he is, getting his private anguish down on paper. Take, if you can, the next seven and a half minutes just to listen – just to listen to this.

Mélancolie
by Francis Poulenc (1899–1963)

17

And here is Francis Poulenc again, writing music during the Nazi occupation of France. On the surface, this is a brief lyrical, improvisatory, neo-romantic pastorale – but the clue is in the title. As befits a man who was depressed by the occupation and at constant risk of persecution for being openly gay, the shadows gradually lengthen over its surface; a tender but potentially crushing beauty hovers in its wings.

Theme from *Schindler's List*
by John Williams (b. 1932)

18

To write a decent film score your music has to touch vast numbers of people in a very particular way. I can't think of a better exemplar than John Williams. His music for *Schindler's List*, which was released in the UK on this day in 1993, incorporates traditional aspects of Jewish music that, irrespective of race, seem to vibrate atavistically in our collective consciousness. In less than five minutes he manages to convey something of the unspeakable tragedy of the Holocaust.

19

Hiraeth
by Grace Williams (1906–1977)

Today we mark the birth of the composer Grace Williams with this atmospheric piece for solo harp. *Hiraeth* is a hard word to translate from the Welsh, but it denotes a sort of nostalgic longing. I think you can hear that quality laced throughout the piece.

20

Handel in the Strand
by Percy Grainger (1882–1961)

There's a lot to be said for the occasional piece of music that simply puts a smile on your face. And here you go, here's one. It's not going to change the world, but I do find it cheering when it accompanies me on any number of domestic tasks – emptying the dishwasher, putting on a load of laundry, sorting the bins, etc.

Cello Sonata in G minor, op. 19
3: Andante
by Sergei Rachmaninov (1873–1943)

21

Discovery of music can come from all sorts of places. In this case, it was a moment in Patrick Gale's lovely 2018 novel *Take Nothing With You*. At one point, Gale's main character Eustace, a young cellist, is learning this piece. Not being able to recall the cello sonata off the top of my head, I went straight online and found it, and listened. I simply could not believe the wrenching beauty of what I was hearing.

Sonata for two pianos in D major, K. 448
2: Andante
by Wolfgang Amadeus Mozart (1756–1791)

22

This is the piece used by the scientists who investigated the phenomenon known as the 'Mozart effect'. They found that listening to this music for just ten minutes each day could sufficiently rewire our brains to make us smarter. The research is freely available online if you feel like diving in. Frankly, I'll take any excuse to listen again.

In many cultures, late winter is traditionally a time for meditation and reflection. Yet sometimes, it can feel quite bleak. How could you garner solace and strength from the season's low light levels, and its short days?

När natten skänker frid – When night confers repose
by Karin Rehnqvist (b. 1957)

23

If you live in the northern hemisphere and the dark days of late February are by any chance getting you down by now, here's a dose of luminous contemporary choral music that might just help. This piece is highly atmospheric, simultaneously evoking the icy climes of the composer's native Scandinavia yet glowing with something akin to fire. It's like the sonic equivalent of a really good whisky: listening to it is a gift.

Spiegel im Spiegel
by Arvo Pärt (b. 1935)

24

It's Estonian Independence Day: a good moment to hear from one of that country's most musical sons, Arvo Pärt. There's a lot more to Pärt's sound world than this glistening reverie but I hope it delivers a moment of stillness and serenity to your day.

25

12 Sonatas, op. 16: Sonata prima
5: Soli violini
by Isabella Leonarda (1620–1704)

To one of the most productive and prolific composers of her time: Isabella Leonarda, who died on this day. The set of gentle sonatas that make up her opus 16, from which this lovely, lyrical movement comes, became, when they appeared in Bologna in 1693, the earliest published instrumental works by a woman. That fact alone, I hope you agree, makes them worth a little celebration.

26

Overture from *L'amant anonyme*
1: Allegro presto
by Joseph Boulogne, Chevalier de Saint-Georges
(1745–1799)

Often dubbed – inevitably, if unimaginatively – 'the Black Mozart', Joseph Boulogne is one of classical music's true trailblazers. Born in Guadeloupe and educated in France, he went on to become a fine dancer, a colonel in Europe's first all-Black army regiment during the French Revolution, and a champion swordsman, one of the biggest fencing stars of the day. This was quite the trajectory, given his background as the son of a slave.

Fantasia in F minor for Piano 4 hands, op. 103
by Franz Schubert (1797–1828)

27

Written in the last year of his tragically short life, and published only after his death, this is Schubert at his most melodically endearing yet quietly sophisticated. The format of the work reflects the vogue in nineteenth-century Europe for 'four-hand' music that enabled social music-making without the need for a second piano; incredibly, for all its complexity and drama, this piece requires only one keyboard.

Ô Abre Alas – Open, wings
by Francisca Edviges Neves 'Chiquinha' Gonzaga (1847–1935)

28

An iconic carnival anthem today, from Brazil's first professional female composer. In her long and vibrant life, Gonzaga produced some two thousand works that helped to put Brazilian classical music on the map; pieces that, in their inventive fusion of European dance forms and Afro-Brazilian rhythms, still sound thrillingly fresh.

29

Overture
from *The Barber of Seville*
by Gioachino Rossini (1792–868)

Rossini was the creator of music so mainstream it might feasibly be described as the pop music of his day. Apparently his catchy melodies were whistled on the streets, and one well-regarded physician in Naples reported over forty cases of women dying of excitement while watching one of his operas. Whether or not you are reading this in a leap year, I hope you'll raise a toast to the anniversary of the birth of one of music's great individuals.

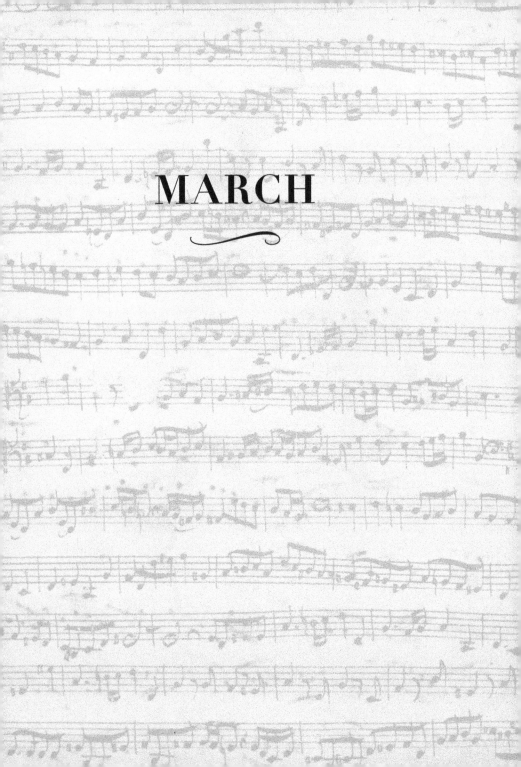

MARCH

Ar hyd y Nos – All through the Night
Traditional Welsh

1

For St David's Day, here's a much loved traditional song, first recorded in the 1784 collection *Musical and Poetical Relicks of the Welsh Bards*, as assembled by the legendary Welsh bard, harpist, poet, composer and arranger Edward Jones (a.k.a. 'Bardd y Brenin'). *Dydd Gŵyl Dewi Hapus!*

Lento
by Aleksey Igudesman (b. 1973)

2

As one half of the musical comedy duo Igudesman & Joo, today's multi-talented composer Aleksey Igudesman has racked up almost sixteen million views on YouTube. As well as being a violinist, conductor, comedian, film-maker, producer, actor, poet and tech entrepreneur, he is also, as today's beautifully meandering, meditative piece proves, a talented composer in his own right.

3

Three Dream Portraits
2: 'Dream Variation'
by Margaret Bonds (1913–1972)

Today we mark the birthday of one of the first Black classical performers to gain recognition in the US. At university, Margaret Bonds experienced terrible racial discrimination, but in the library one day she found a poem by Langston Hughes, 'The Negro Speaks of Rivers', which helped give her a sense of security. She later befriended Hughes and collaborated with him on many projects, including the song collection *Three Dream Portraits*, of which this fabulous setting is the second part.

4

Concerto for two trumpets in C major, RV 537
1: Allegro
by Antonio Vivaldi (1678–1741)

The mighty Antonio Vivaldi, one of the all-time musical greats, was born on this day: we shall celebrate with some sparkling double trumpets. I love the bright, fanfare-like opening for this concerto and the call-and-response exchange he creates between both the solo lines and the ensemble.

Symphony no. 1 in D major, op. 25 ('Classical')
1: Allegro
by Sergei Prokofiev (1891–1953)

5

Always a bit of a renegade spirit, Prokofiev, who died on this day, is doing something really interesting here – writing an almost satirical pastiche of a 'Classical' symphony from the vantage point of 1917, the year of the Russian Revolution, when all around him established aesthetic forms (not to mention whole nations, empires) were fragmenting and falling apart. He wrote this cheering, cheeky symphony at the age of twenty-six, whilst on holiday.

Sonata for violin and piano no. 5 in F major, op. 24 ('Spring')
1: Allegro
by Ludwig van Beethoven (1770–1827)

6

It was not Beethoven himself who dubbed this piece the 'Spring Sonata'; that nickname was applied many years later, after his death. But, my goodness, is it appropriate! This is music as joyous and fresh and life-affirming as you can get. Wherever you are in the world, and whether or not spring has yet sprung round your way, I hope you feel newly awakened and energized by this amazing music.

7

'Morning on the Limpopo; Matlou Women' from *Limpopo Songs* by Paola Prestini (b. 1975)

Paola Prestini is a force of nature: an accomplished composer who has shaken up the contemporary classical scene in the US. In recent years she has launched National Sawdust, a performing arts space in Brooklyn that is also a hub for curation, criticism, recordings and vital initiatives such as the annual Hildegard competition for composers who identify as female, trans or non-binary. She is a boundary-pusher, a generous spirit who represents, for the classical world, a proper breath of fresh air.

8

Prelude, op. 73 by Mana-Zucca Cassel (1885–1981)

Today is International Women's Day and, it happens, the day that one inordinately talented musical woman died. This fabulous female was much in demand as an international piano soloist, but also starred in several musical comedies, appearing on Broadway as an actress and singer, and writing the smash hit song 'I Love Life' . . . all the while being drawn to compose wonderfully textured classical pieces like this prelude which, I hope you will agree, is a true delight.

Reflecting on International Women's Day, take a moment to consider and celebrate the intrepid and pioneering female musicians that you have most been inspired by in your life.

9

Abendlied – Evening Song
by Josef Rheinberger (1839–1901)

It goes without saying that this is a piece that could be enjoyed at any time of day, but, if you can, I would recommend that you take four and a half minutes, on this or any evening, to listen to this serene, supremely peaceful work. For me it always sets the day just passed in a different light, and I'm invariably grateful for that change in perspective.

10

Zigeunerweisen, op. 20
by Pablo de Sarasate (1844–1908)

As a fiddle player myself, I sometimes fantasize about what it must have been like to see some of the great violinists of history in action: Fritz Kreisler, Joseph Joachim, Niccolò Paganini, Marie Hall, Jascha Heifetz and Pablo de Sarasate, who was born on this day. Celebrated for his virtuosic technique as a performer, he composed pieces of great stylistic panache that are as exhilarating to listen to as they are hair-raising to play.

History of Tango
2: 'Café 1930'
by Astor Piazzolla (1921–1992)

11

Another musical birthday to celebrate today, that of the Argentine tango master Astor Piazzolla who, as well as being synonymous with the dance traditions of his homeland, was also steeped in classical music. This piece comes from Piazzolla's seminal work *History of Tango*. As far as I'm concerned, a piece such as this is another powerful argument against the policing of musical genre boundaries at all.

Miserere in C minor
by Jan Dismas Zelenka (1679–1745)

12

In his day, Zelenka was greatly admired. Telemann, for example, was so in awe of his abilities that he was drawn into a complex plot to try and steal copies of his work. J. S. Bach, meanwhile, tirelessly lobbied Zelenka's employers to get an appointment at the same court, just to be closer to his hero. Zelenka is hardly ever heard today, which just goes to show what a fickle old thing history can be.

13

The Road Home
by Stephen Paulus (1949–2014)

In 2001, American composer Stephen Paulus was commissioned by a choir asking for a short 'folk'-type choral arrangement. He discovered a tune called 'The Lone Wild Bird' in *The Southern Harmony Songbook* of 1835. The melody is built on a scale called the 'pentatonic' that has existed for centuries in all musical cultures around the world; in other words, it is one of humanity's most common and unifying musical expressions.

14

Tarantella: 'La Carpinese'
Traditional

Doing the tarantella has been a custom in Southern Europe for centuries, allegedly since the villagers in the Italian seaside port of Taranto discovered that a certain kind of whirling, high-octane dance could act as an antidote to the deadly bite of the local 'tarantula' spider. Magical antidotal properties aside, the tarantella invariably makes for an adrenaline-pumping listen.

*We're approaching the Spring Equinox. How will you embrace
this period of hope, change and new beginnings? Are you feeling
more energized as the light returns? Are you noticing new things
as the seasons change? Try to see the world in a new light,
literally and figuratively . . .*

15

Reflets – Reflections
by Lili Boulanger (1893–1918)

It was on this day in 1918 that the music world lost one of its most promising talents. Lili Boulanger was only twenty-four when her life was claimed by intestinal tuberculosis, or what we would now term Crohn's Disease. When she died she left behind instrumental works, choral pieces, an unfinished opera, and a handful of songs, including this dark but radiant setting of words by Maurice Maeterlinck.

16

Salve regina in C Minor
1: 'Salve regina'
by Giovanni Battista Pergolesi (1710–1736)

Speaking of musical lives cut drastically short, today we mark the death from tuberculosis of an Italian Baroque genius. This would have been among the very last music that Pergolesi wrote, before the 26-year-old died in abject poverty. I find it heart-wrenchingly exquisite music; the knowledge that it was composed by a human being at the very close of a life that should, if things were just, have continued for many more decades, only makes it more moving.

Lorica of St Patrick
by Charles Villiers Stanford (1852–1924)

17

With words attributed to St Patrick (372–466) and his Irish ministry from the fifth century, this seems a fitting work for today, St Patrick's Day. Written in the style of a Druid's incantation, it's a prayer of protection for anyone who faces a long journey, invoking layer upon layer of blessings. The Dublin-born Stanford took the words and worked them into his own arrangement of an old melody from the Ancient Irish Church; the effect, I think, is beautiful.

Miocheries, op. 126 no. 13
'La toute petite s'endort' – 'The littlest falls asleep'
by Mel Bonis (1858–1937)

18

It twists my heart, listening to Mel Bonis's very beautiful but also quietly devastating take on the *berceuse*, or lullaby, especially on this date. She died on this day, having never got over the death of her beloved younger son, five years previously.

19

Four Studies
3: 'Slow Canons'
by Nico Muhly (b. 1981)

In this arresting and intriguing piece, the New York-based Nico Muhly employs the device of a musical drone – a technique which has existed, in many different musical cultures, for centuries – and intricately laces two minimalist solo violin lines around it to create a luminous and eerie soundscape. It's only a few minutes long but unlike anything I've heard.

20

Zefiro torna e di soavi accenti – Return, O Zephyr
by Claudio Monteverdi (1567–1643)

Monteverdi's settings of madrigals – secular songs for multiple voices – are filled with surprises, with dynamic ups and downs and moments of such spontaneity and naturalness that we take for granted now what would have sounded impossibly new in his day.

This one is a classic. Monteverdi sets a rhapsodic ode to spring by the poet Ottavio Rinuccini, in a work celebrating the bountiful promise of the season. As ever with Monteverdi, the music serves its text with infectious exuberance.

Vergnugte Ruh', beliebte Seelenlust – Delightful rest, beloved pleasure of the soul, BWV 170
1: Aria
by Johann Sebastian Bach (1685–1750)

21

Depending on whether you're consulting the old (Julian) or new (Gregorian) calendar, J. S. Bach was either born today, or on 31 March. What to say about him that can possibly be sufficiently captured in mere words? For me, speaking as a confused agnostic, Bach is quite simply the closest I come to the divine. When nothing makes sense, or when everything makes sense, there's Bach. Happy birthday to the greatest.

Recomposed: Vivaldi Four Seasons
'Spring 3'
by Max Richter (b. 1966)

22

We have another birthday today: that of one of contemporary music's towering minds. Max Richter is a synthesizer of all that he hears around him, soaking up influences from a rich variety of sources. And yet everything he writes has its own distinctive essence. In today's piece, Richter pays homage to Antonio Vivaldi. Taken from his phenomenal 2012 reworking of *The Four Seasons*, this 'Spring section' is three minutes of astonishing music that floors me every single time I hear it.

Make a classical playlist for your next social gathering.
Notice the mood of the evening and how your guests respond.
Were you surprised by their reactions?

Heal You
by Anna Meredith (b. 1978)

As well as opera, vocal, orchestral and instrumental music, Anna Meredith has turned her fierce intelligence and playful imagination to beatboxer symphonies, pop music and film scores. Her music has been performed everywhere from the hallowed Royal Albert Hall during The Last Night of the Proms to a service station off the M6 (in a particularly memorable body-percussion flash-mob performance). This short, evocative choral piece sets words by the storyteller Philip Ridley and is a real mind-cleanser, in the best possible way.

Viola Concerto in G major
1: Largo
by Georg Philip Telemann (1681–1767)

Telemann in a mellow mood today, his birthday, writing for the instrument that some say is closest to the human voice (and others are just mean about; the viola having long been the butt of orchestral jokes). Of the seventy-eight instrumental concertos that this hugely prolific composer wrote, this is the one for which he's best known.

25

3 Hungarian Folksongs from Csík, BB 45b
1: Rubato
by Béla Bartók (1881–1945)

Today we commemorate the birth of the man who would not only become the leading Hungarian composer of his day, but one of the most important and pioneering collectors of folk song in musical history. In 1907 Béla Bartók set off for the Eastern Carpathian mountains with a mission to listen to, record and gather folk music. The trip was incredibly fruitful, and among the countless melodies he picked up were three simple tunes played to him on a peasant flute, which he duly set for piano.

26

12 Notations pour piano, arranged for orchestra
1: Fantasque – Modéré
by Pierre Boulez (1925–2016)

Pierre Boulez, who was born on this day, was all about creating 'different feelings' in musical textures, sounds and time. Even as a young man Boulez exhibited absolute certainty about what he wanted the future of music to sound like – and suffice to say, it was like nothing that had been before.

'Bevo al tuo fresco sorriso' – 'I drink to your intoxicating smile'
from *La Rondine*
by Giacomo Puccini (1858–1924)

27

Today we revel in a straight-up unabashed love song, opera-style, with a gorgeous moment from Puccini's opera *La Rondine* (*The Swallow*), which was premiered in Monte Carlo on this day in 1917. As two couples come together towards the end of one of opera's least overblown plots they raise a toast which I think we can all get behind: *Let us drink to love!*

10 Preludes, op. 23
No. 10 in G flat major: Largo
by Sergei Rachmaninov (1873–1943)

28

A hauntingly lovely piece, marking the death on this day of one of music's all-time greats, Sergei Rachmaninov. The phenomenal Russian composer and pianist was experiencing financial difficulty when he holed up in a Moscow hotel to write the set of preludes from which this closing movement comes. But if the motivation to produce this music was largely driven by financial necessity, in no way is the art compromised.

Where do you most like to listen to music? Can you think about why that is? Could you perhaps try a new setting for your listening, and note any positive differences?

Waltz
from *Eugene Onegin*
by Pyotr Ilyich Tchaikovsky (1840–1893)

29

After yesterday's Rachmaninov, today a cheery and uplifting waltz by one of the composers who was most directly influential to him. It was on this day in 1879 that Tchaikovsky's magnificent take on Pushkin's verse-novel *Eugene Onegin* was premiered. Tchaikovsky was unashamedly sympathetic towards his heroine, and openly scornful of the 'cad' Onegin who rejects her; in many ways he wears his own highly emotional heart on his sleeve, which is why the music packs such a punch.

Ave generosa
by Hildegard of Bingen (c. 1098–1179)

30

To one of the most extraordinary figures from the Medieval era today, the polymathic Christian visionary, medic, writer, poet, composer and very early feminist Hildegard of Bingen. Her music is characterized by an almost improvisatory melodic freedom, creating an ethereal sound world that points far forward into the distant future; it is perhaps this that gives her compositions such a sense of timelessness.

31

Herr, gehe nicht ins Gericht – Lord, do not pass judgement on your servant, Cantata BWV 105
3: Aria: 'Wie zittern und wanken Der Sünder Gedanken'
– 'How the thoughts of the sinner tremble and waver'
by Johann Sebastian Bach (1685–1750)

An unapologetic second celebration of Bach's birthday today (see also 21 March). Here he is, a man wrought through with the divine – but also defiantly and gloriously human. A man who loved and lost and laughed and had friends and made mistakes and picked himself up and went on, as we all do. It might sound crazy, but I think one of the things I love most about Bach's music is how non-judgmental, how tolerant, it somehow is. Happy birthday again, my hero.

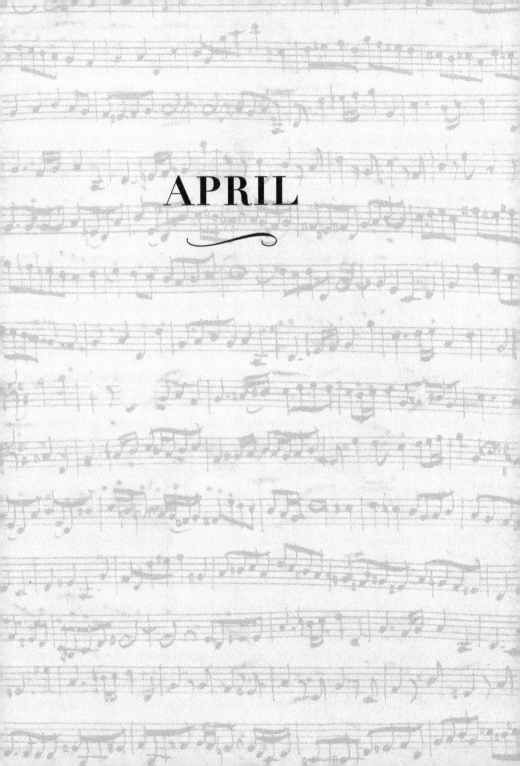

APRIL

Nautilus
by Anna Meredith (b. 1978)

1

Fresh fanfare beats for a brand new month today from one of British music's brightest lights, the Scottish-born Anna Meredith MBE. A former Composer-in-Residence with the BBC Scottish Symphony Orchestra, Meredith's magnificently distinctive work has been performed everywhere from the BBC *Proms* to the 2012 Cultural Olympiad.

Alma redemptoris mater
by Dobrinka Tabakova (b. 1980)

2

After Anna Meredith yesterday, today we hear from another outstanding contemporary voice in British music, the Grammy-nominated composer Dobrinka Tabakova, and her setting of the timeless Marian hymn *Alma redemptoris mater* (we heard Palestrina's back in February).

3

Piano Quintet in F sharp minor, op. 67
3: Allegro agitato – Adagio coma prima – Presto
by Amy Beach (1867–1944)

The largely self-taught Amy Beach's music has its own distinct language, even as it incorporates aspects of the Romanticism of the preceding era and the European composers she held in such high esteem, including Brahms. Far from conservative, even if it doesn't exactly push formal boundaries, her music brims with an energy and sincerity that I find hugely appealing.

4

Symphony no. 3 ('Symphony of Sorrowful Songs')
2: Lento e largo – Tranquillissimo
by Henryk Górecki (1933–2010)

Górecki's Third Symphony, which received its premiere on this day in 1977, has gone on to sell over a million copies. A highly unusual work, it asks us to look tragedy directly in the eye. In each movement, a solo soprano sings a Polish text. This middle movement sets the words of a prayer inscribed by an eighteen-year-old girl on the wall of a Gestapo prison in 1944. The work is all the more moving for the fact that Górecki had lost members of his own family in concentration camps.

*We are just over a quarter of the way through the year.
Acknowledging that time is linear, in what ways can you express
your gratitude for its passage? After all: you are still here! Who are
the people you feel most grateful to? How might you try and
express that to them?*

5

Pavane pour une infante défunte – Pavane for a Dead Princess by Maurice Ravel (1875–1937)

I sometimes wonder what it must have been like, to have been sitting in the audience at the Société Nationale de Musique concert in Paris on this day in 1902, and to hear this extraordinary music unfold, note by note, for the very first time in public. What a gift!

6

More sweet than my refrain by Howard Skempton (b. 1947)

A tender vocal miniature today from one of Britain's greatest contemporary composers, laying aside his usual adventures in experimentalism to set a radiant fragment by Ralph Waldo Emerson, the great American poet who celebrated the existence of the sublime in both humanity and nature.

Night Bird
by Karen Tanaka (b. 1961)

7

Happy birthday to Karen Tanaka, one of Japan's leading contemporary composers. This might sound crazy, but I find listening to this piece is like stepping over a threshold and falling into some sort of other dimension. It's so incredibly eerie and beautiful, with the mournful lines of the alto saxophone offset by an otherworldly backdrop of electronics and gentle percussion effects.

Berceuse in D flat major, op. 57
by Frédéric Chopin (1810–1849)

8

In the spring of 1917, the poet Edward Thomas spent ten weeks in France, where he kept a war diary. One of his men had brought a gramophone to the Western Front and Thomas would make a note of what music they heard each day. One of the pieces they played was this piano lullaby. 8 April 1917 would be Edward Thomas's last day on this earth. He was killed fighting in the Battle of Arras the very next day. I like to imagine the possible consolation that he might have drawn from this music in the days leading up to his futile death.

9

En la Macarenita
Traditional, arranged by Bob Chilcott (b. 1955)

For something completely different today, we say happy birthday to one of British choral music's contemporary heroes, Bob Chilcott. Here's his take on a traditional Spanish folk song – in which a girl heads down to the Macarena and catches the wooing eyes of a dancing stranger . . .

10

The Lamentations of Jeremiah the Prophet:
Lamentations for Holy Wednesday
Lamentatio 1
by Jan Dismas Zelenka (1679–1745)

Today we travel back to the era of Bohemian Baroque and a composer whose harmonic innovations, structural daring and dazzling way with counterpoint have been almost entirely – and I would argue, unfairly – forgotten. This piece is almost thirteen minutes long, but it unfolds with such sustained drama, via such crunchy dissonances and such blissful resolutions, that I find it always rewards a listen handsomely.

Music has the ability to transport us across land and seas and even back in time. What period of time would you most like to go back to and visit? Close your eyes and see where the music takes you . . .

11

Tres piezas, op. 6
1: 'Cuyana'
by Alberto Ginastera (1916–1983)

No matter how many times I hear this atmospheric solo piano piece, I never quite know what's coming next – in the best possible way. I love how the composer takes us on a meandering melodic journey and just at the moment when you feel you know exactly where you are, he picks you up and deposits you somewhere else, somewhere completely unexpected.

12

Metamorphosen
by Richard Strauss (1864–1949)

On this day in 1945, Richard Strauss completed his emotionally searing work for twenty-three strings, Metamorphosen, towards the end of World War Two and just a few years before his death. In the dejection it enacts, the intensity of the feelings it evokes, this piece for me distils some quintessence of universal human loss and never leaves me anything other than utterly shaken.

It is a singularly moving musical response to the senselessness of war – any war.

Piano Trio in D major, op. 1
1: Allegro non troppo, con espressione
by Erich Wolfgang Korngold (1897–1957)

13

The publication in 1910 of this piece stunned the musical world at the time, written as it was by a thirteen-year-old boy. Korngold would go on to have a stellar career in opera and Hollywood, writing some of the most iconic movie scores of the era. I think those gifts for narrative and finely honed dramatic instincts are all on display in this first published work, which he sweetly dedicated to his father.

Avril 14th
by Richard D. James, aka Aphex Twin (b. 1971)
arr. Christian Badzura (b. 1977)

14

And breathe. This simple, lullaby-like piece has an instantly restorative effect on me. Originally written for piano, it also works a treat when arranged for violin.

Reflect on the music you've enjoyed throughout your life. Has your relationship to music changed as you've become older? Does it change depending on how you are feeling? How does your mood and body respond to different music? Can you detect any particular patterns?

Partita for 8 voices
2: Sarabande
by Caroline Shaw (b. 1982)

15

It was on this day in 2013 that the American composer Caroline Shaw became the youngest ever winner of the Pulitzer Prize for Music, for the *Partita* from which this movement comes. This fantastically original work references everything from Georgian male voice vocal traditions to Korean *p'ansori* singing; it is unlike anything I have ever heard. I hope you'll simply open your ears and your hearts to its strange and wonderful power.

Magnolia
Part 1, no. 1: 'Magnolias'
by R. Nathaniel Dett (1882–1943)

16

A spray of musical magnolia today, courtesy of the Canadian–American composer (Robert) Nathaniel Dett, who descended from escaped slaves, and became, in 1908, the first Black student to complete the Bachelor of Music degree at Oberlin Conservatory. I find that whatever state I'm in, its aura of freshness and rebirth – complete with a quick April shower in the middle – cannot fail to improve my mood. Consider it a three-and-a-half-minute dose of musical springtime.

17

Ellis Island
by Meredith Monk (b. 1942)

When Meredith Monk was invited to make a film about Ellis Island, which had been the iconic point of entry for millions of immigrants to the USA, she applied her characteristically imaginative and original vision to the process, weaving documentary material around contemporary images and writing an evocative and atmospheric soundtrack.

18

Stabat mater
7: 'Eia mater, fons amoris' – 'Oh mother, fount of love'
by Antonio Vivaldi (1678–1741)

The thirteenth-century text *Stabat mater doloroso* is a deeply moving meditation on the crucifixion of a beloved child. Vivaldi sets the work in nine parts, of which this wrenching movement is the seventh. I found this piece deeply moving *before* I had a child; these days, it's liable to reduce me to a sobbing wreck. Yet, in the way of the greatest music, its beauty is somehow, simultaneously, its own redemption.

Valse lente – slow waltz
by Germaine Tailleferre (1892–1983)

19

There is a terrific picture of Germaine Tailleferre standing amid a cluster of male composers and everything in her expression, her demeanour, says, 'Yeah? And what?' Born on this day, Tailleferre was not someone to let her gender stand in the way of anything. Through the twentieth century's many shifts in musical style, she held her nerve and navigated her own distinct path.

'Music for a while'
from *Oedipus*
by Henry Purcell (1659–1695)

20

Purcell is one of the most important musicians England has ever produced, and his reach over modern music remains profound. You can also hear his harmonies, his bold suspensions and resolutions, and his formal structures – such as the ascending 'ground bass' that underpins this piece – reimagined and reanimated not just in later classical compositions but in modern pop songs and film soundtracks galore.

*Close your eyes and ground yourself in the emotion that comes up
in you, whatever it is. Do you find yourself wanting to move?
Or maybe it's the opposite; maybe you feel internally quiet,
even stilled? Let the music take over, release any resistance,
and notice how you truthfully respond.*

Messe de Nostre Dame
1. Kyrie
by Guillaume de Machaut (c. 1300–1377)

21

When I think of the immeasurable musical significance of the Mass in Western culture, with all the towering examples that would follow, from Bach to Mozart to Beethoven to Bruckner to Dvořák, it sends shivers down my spine to think that this is the *very first one.*

Danza gaya
by Madeleine Dring (1923–1977)

22

Madeleine Dring's style is refreshingly unpretentious – impressive for a woman trying to make her voice heard in a landscape still overwhelmingly dominated by men. I imagine she must have been under considerable pressure to do something 'different', but instead she sticks to her guns and writes pieces of rhythmic vibrancy and great charm. This is not music that's going to change the world, but if it doesn't set your toes tapping I'll eat my hat.

23

'How Sweet the Moonlight'
from *The Merchant of Venice*
by Jocelyn Pook (b.1960)

Composers throughout the centuries have been drawn to the words of Shakespeare, who was born and died on this day, and more recently to Shakespeare on celluloid. Jocelyn Pook's score for *The Merchant of Venice* (2004), which starred Al Pacino and Jeremy Irons, manages to capture the atmosphere of early Renaissance music yet gives it a modern twist. Her setting of the luscious poetry of Act 5, scene 1 creates a particularly atmospheric mood.

24

'Curtain Tune'
from *The Tempest*
by Matthew Locke (1621–1677)

Okay, I couldn't resist. More Shakespeare. This time from the man who was arguably the leading composer for the stage of his era, and music for a 1674 production of an opera version of *The Tempest*. The 'Curtain Tune' depicts the fateful shipwreck from which the rest of the plot emerges, and is full of engaging musical twists and turns.

Keltic Suite, op. 29
2: 'Lament'
by John Foulds (1880–1939)

25

This piece is unashamedly romantic, encapsulating a certain essential British nostalgia which has proved enduringly popular. I listen and I can't help but see rolling hills, perhaps a train journey, steam rising off a cup of tea – yet it manages not to curdle into cliché.

Anthracite Fields
4: 'Flowers'
by Julia Wolfe (b. 1958)

26

Premiered in Philadelphia on this day in 2014, the Pulitzer Prize-winning oratorio *Anthracite Fields* evokes Pennsylvania coal-mining life around the turn of the twentieth century. Small but revealing details abound. Julia Wolfe heard that women in the small mining villages would try to bring a degree of colour and joy to their impoverished existences using flowers. She builds on that image, having the chorus sing a list of those flowers during this section, and it is so moving and powerful.

While you listen to the music, take a moment to check in with your physical body. How are you sitting? How do your eyes feel? Or your jaw, your lower back, your feet? Are there areas you can adjust or relax, for more comfort? Try incorporating this practice daily.

Romance
by Alexander Scriabin (1871–1915)

Music by the Russian composer Scriabin today, a very unusual figure for his time. He was a mystic, much intrigued by the possibilities of musical symbolism, Gnosticism and theosophy, and his work is laced with these ideas throughout. I hope you'll agree it's a work of tender and searching beauty.

Five Songs, op. 105
1: 'Wie Melodien zieht es mir' – 'It moves like a melody'
by Johannes Brahms (1833–1897)
arr. Jascha Heifetz (1901–1987)

This song is the sort of piece I might turn to when I need a quick sonic fix: a little over three minutes of purely lovely music. Sometimes, I find, that's enough; that's more than enough.

29

Black, Brown and Beige Suite
1: Introduction
by Duke Ellington (1899–1974)
arr. Nigel Kennedy (b. 1956)

I once asked my former BBC Radio 3 colleague Rob Cowan, who in his view was the greatest composer of the twentieth century. He answered: Duke Ellington. This might come as a surprise, given Ellington's reputation as the king of jazz, but for Ellington himself there were only two types of music: 'good' and 'bad'. It goes without saying that he composed, across some two thousand pieces, a hell of a lot of good.

30

Songs Without Words
2: 'Lied' – 'Song'
by Anne Cawrse (b. 1981)

Born in rural South Australia, to a non-musical farming family, Anne Cawrse composes music with unpretentious intelligence and a beguiling directness. Very rarely programmed outside of her own country – yet! – I reckon she deserves a wider audience.

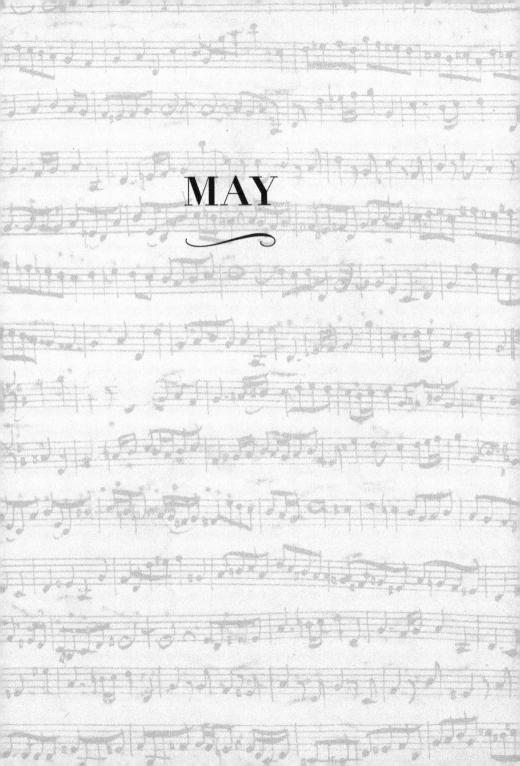

MAY

From the Bohemian Forest, op. 68 B. 133
5: 'Waldesruhe' – 'Silent Woods'
by Antonín Dvořák (1841–1904)
arr. Lothar Niefind and Gunter Ribke

1

I don't generally press my readers to listen to a certain arrangement of a piece, but today I am making an exception. This particular modern arrangement for solo cello and cello ensemble is utterly charming. It's five and a half minutes of romance without a cliché in sight. I find it hopelessly touching. Especially when I listen to it today, the day that Dvořák died.

Concerto for recorder and two violins in A minor
2: Largo
by Alessandro Scarlatti (1660–1725)

2

Today we enjoy a two-minute sliver of Baroque beauty from a composer whose achievements have often been overlooked for those of his brilliant son Domenico. But Scarlatti *père* clearly had a great knack for a good theme, and his formal innovations and use of chromatic harmony was prescient, prefiguring much of what was to come in the future Classical and Romantic eras.

3

Rosary Sonata no. 16 in G Minor for solo violin
Passacaglia
by Heinrich Ignaz Franz von Biber (1644–1704)

Technically fiendish, abounding in outrageously demanding multi-string chords, this piece requires of its player great heart, or it can come across as rather cold and mathematical. Played well, though, with the right balance of virtuosity and soul, I find its spare, clear lines have the effect of a mental detox; I listen and it's as though my brain is somehow re-wired. Incredible.

4

L'Ondine
by Cecile Chaminade (1857–1944)

Published in 1900, this glittlering little tone-sketch for solo piano depicts a water sprite, deftly rendered with fluid arpeggios (broken chords) and rippling pianistic effects that have a pianist traversing the whole keyboard.

The Yellow Cake Revue
3. 'Farewell to Stromness'
by Peter Maxwell Davies (1934–2016)

5

In 1971 composer Peter Maxwell Davies moved to Orkney. Towards the end of that decade, he became aware that the South of Scotland Electricity Board was intending to mine Yellowcake uranium deposits near Stromness, a town on the largest island, to fuel a nuclear power plant. Maxwell Davies poured his objections into a unique work of art, comprising cabaret-style songs and recitations as well as a pair of piano interludes. It was premiered on this day in 1990 and has been beloved ever since.

The Lark
by Mikhail Glinka (1804–1857)
arr. Mily Balakirev (1837–1910)

6

This piece was originally a song, part of a twelve-part collection called *Farewell to St Petersburg*, and although it's lovely in that version, it's the subsequent arrangement for solo piano by Glinka's young acolyte, Mily Balakirev, that I fell in love with the first time I heard it. Both wistful and wandering, birdlike indeed, with a piano melody that, at times, seems to take radiant flight.

Music can provide consolation and reassurance. Think about – and try to describe – a memorable place where you felt happy and safe. Write down the memory. Maybe music can help to access the same sense of safety or ease?

Violin Sonata no. 1 in G major, op. 78
1: Vivace ma no troppo
by Johannes Brahms (1833–1897)

7

Today we hear from Johannes Brahms, who was born on this day
– and a piece that always feels to me like the sun coming out in
musical form. Though prolific, Brahms was ruthlessly self-critical
and unforgiving: he tore up at least four violin sonatas that did not
survive in the process of creating the three that do. While part of me
regrets this, greedily wishing he'd written more, you just can't argue
with the ones he left behind.

Spitfire Prelude & Fugue
1: Prelude
by William Walton (1902–1983)

8

It was on this date in 1945 that the Allies of World War Two formally
accepted Nazi Germany's unconditional surrender of its armed
forces, so I thought we could indulge, on VE Day, in a wartime
classic. William Walton was exempted from military service by the
British government on the condition he compose music for their
morale-boosting propaganda films. Right from the opening brass
fanfare in this iconic piece, he delivers the goods.

9

Act 1 'letter scene'
from *Eugene Onegin*
by Pyotr Ilyich Tchaikovsky (1840–1893)

I was fifteen and had just been dumped by the first great love of my life. A few nights later I got dragged to see *Eugene Onegin*. I was wretched with heartbreak and barely paying attention. But then – wait – I'm watching a girl pull out a piece of paper and start to sing. And now she's writing a letter, to this man who has heartlessly crushed her love, and it's so beautiful, and I can't help but be transfixed. And now I get it, why opera – for all its ridiculousness – can sometimes be the very truest and most powerful art form there is.

10

Merry Christmas, Mr Lawrence
by Ryuichi Sakamoto (b. 1952)

It was on this day in 1983 that the Japanese war movie *Merry Christmas, Mr Lawrence* was premiered. It marked a major debut (as both actor and composer) for Ryuichi Sakamoto, who has since gone on to win an Oscar, a BAFTA, a Grammy and two Golden Globes for his music.

The first time I heard this piece, I had to immediately stop what I was doing to find out what it was. And once I knew, I took it into my heart and I listened to it again and again and again. I hope you will too.

Symphony no. 1 ('Afro–American')
4: 'Aspiration': Lento, con risoluzione
by William Grant Still (1895–1978)

11

This has the dubious honour of being the first symphony written by an African–American to be performed by a major American orchestra. I say 'dubious' because that event took place in 1931, which, by any measure, is depressingly, outrageously late. Still's legacy is remarkable: he was the first Black man to conduct a leading American orchestra, the first to have an opera performed by a major company, the first to have his opera performed on national television, and so on. His name should be known by every classical fan.

Three Melodies, op. 7
1: 'Après un rêve' – 'After a Dream'
by Gabriel Fauré (1845–1924)

12

Today marks the anniversary of the birth of one of French music's great innovators and influencers, Gabriel Fauré, who represents a vital bridge between the end of the Romantic era and the advent of early-twentieth-century Modernism. Composer of orchestral works, choral music and one of the great Requiem settings of all time, he also produced miniatures such as this which are perfect little gems of the repertoire.

13

Twilight
by Arthur Sullivan (1842–1900)

Yesterday we were in Fauré's dream world, and we remain in a somewhere nocturnal state today with this piece by Arthur Sullivan (as in Gilbert & Sullivan). Sullivan, who was born on this day, contributed an inestimable amount to the English musical scene, yet often infuriated classical critics for writing music that was – shock horror! – widely accessible. Without question his was music for the people, in the very best possible sense.

14

6 Mélodies, op. 5
No. 3 in E flat major: Andante soave
by Fanny Mendelssohn (1805–1847)

When I listen to this lovely piece, I can't help but picture Fanny – perhaps sitting at home at her keyboard, dreaming about her brother off on his grand tour around Europe while she was forced to stay at home and wait to get married. I hear a young, brilliant woman pouring her curiosity and her intelligence and her empathy into outstandingly good music that would remain neglected and underrated for the best part of another 150 years, and still has to fight to be heard.

Do you have any regrets from this year? Note them down and consider what you would have done differently. Try to make amends; then exercise self-compassion and radical forgiveness. Try to move on. As the lives of so many of these composers show, very little is within our control, except how we respond to things life throws our way.

15

Lamento della ninfa – The Nymph's Lament
from Madrigals, Book 8
4: 'Amor'
by Claudio Monteverdi (1567–1643)

Monteverdi, who was baptized on this day, was really the earliest major composer to clock that a human being singing a single vocal line could be a very, very powerful thing. It sounds so obvious now, but from that simple revelation comes opera, comes lieder, comes bel canto concert arias, and comes, obviously, the modern pop song as we know it. He quarried the rock from which every subsequent vocal sculpture has come, and aren't we thankful for it?

16

Valse élégiaque
by Valborg Aulin (1860–1928)

I discovered this lovely lilting waltz fairly recently on an album called *Neglected Works for Piano*. Confession time: I had never heard of today's composer. For me it's always a bittersweet feeling, a story such as this. On the one hand, it makes me happy that we're finally rediscovering a totally neglected composer; on the other hand, it serves as a painful reminder of how many other forgotten female voices there must be, scattered throughout history.

Lyric Pieces Book 5, op. 54
No. 4: Notturno
by Edvard Grieg (1843–1907)

17

Today is Norway Day, and it is to the ultimate poster-boy for Norwegian classical music that we turn. Edvard Grieg's *Lyric Pieces* do rather brilliantly what it says on the tin. Poetic, folksy, nostalgic without ever being cloying, they are among the most charming miniatures of the nineteenth-century piano literature: the perfect quick classical fix.

'Der Trunkene im Frühling' – 'The Drunkard in Spring'
from *Das Lied von der Erde – The Song of the Earth*
by Gustav Mahler (1860–1911)

18

The epic song cycle *Das Lied von der Erde* is often described as Gustav Mahler's greatest 'symphony'; alas the composer, who died on this day in 1911, did not live to hear it performed.

19

Symphony no. 1 in C minor
4: Allegro maestoso
by Alice Mary Smith (1839–1884)

Women in the nineteenth century almost invariably stuck to forms considered just about respectable for 'lady-composers', such as art songs, chamber works or piano miniatures. Not so the heroic Alice Mary Smith, who was born on this day. This vibrant piece, composed when Smith was just twenty-four, carries the estimable title of being the first symphony ever written by a British woman. Strong work, sister.

20

Scherzo no. 2 in C minor, op. 14
by Clara Schumann (1819–1896)

Clara Schumann, who died on this day, was a force of nature. There was seemingly nothing she couldn't do: she was as accomplished a pianist as Liszt; as gifted a composer as her husband Robert; as impressive a wife, mother, grandmother and general show-on-the-road keeper as I've come across, past or present. That she achieved what she did in the face of such adversity – from her over-protective father, from society, from Robert's devastating mental illness – is all the more astonishing.

Which pieces of music have been bringing you the most joy lately?
Make a note, and even a playlist, so you can return to them
when you need a moment of comfort.

21

Fratres
by Arvo Pärt (b. 1935)

Pärt has helped us change how we hear music; he developed a distinctive and influential musical language based on Medieval musical principles and this piece emerged as a direct result. Composed in 1977, *Fratres* (meaning 'brothers') is based around a set of variations and recurring motifs, all spinning into a mesmerizing, meditative whole.

22

Requiem Mass
7: Libera me
by Giuseppe Verdi (1813–1901)

It truly sends shivers down my spine to think that, on this day in 1874, at the San Marco church in Milan, a group of singers and musicians came together, under the direction of the composer himself, and out of the silence in that church, the first notes of this extraordinary piece emerged. Maybe it sounds crazy, but this fact moves me so: that one day, this music did not exist, lay silent as black marks on a page, and that then it did. And will, now, for ever.

Phantasy Trio
by Joan Trimble (1915–2000)

23

Along with her sister Valerie, a fellow pianist with whom she put on fantastically popular duet recitals, the Irish composer Joan Trimble was practically a household name in the 1940s and 1950s. She is not someone we hear much about these days, yet she was clearly a force of nature. I always find this piece intensely atmospheric, a sonic soundscape I can lose myself in completely.

Piano Concerto no. 5 in E flat major, op. 73 ('Emperor')
1: Allegro
by Ludwig van Beethoven (1770–1827)

24

Beethoven's final piano concerto is a colossus, no other word for it. He catapults the soloist into the action, with just a single chord of support from the orchestra, and basically cries, 'Let's go!' I can think of few more thrilling musical rides.

25

Milonga
by Jorge Cardoso (b. 1949)

Today is Argentina Day, so I've chosen music by one of that country's leading contemporary classical composers. A multi-talented musician, Cardoso is a guitarist, composer, teacher and prolific author – as well as a qualified medical doctor. (Seriously.)

A '*milonga*' is a place or a gathering where people go to dance the tango; it may also mean a particular type of dance or a particular tune to which *tangueros* dance.

26

Aether
by Hildur Guðnadóttir (b. 1982)

To a contemporary musical powerhouse today, the classically-trained but genre-fluid Icelandic composer Hildur Guðnadóttir. Her profoundly ruminative works often call for a wide range of textures and instrumentation, but this is an early solo piece from her 2009 album *Without Sinking*. I find a gleaming luminosity at the core of all Guðnadóttir's music.

Caprice in E major, op. 1 no. 1
by Niccolò Paganini (1782–1840)

27

Today we celebrate the legacy of one of the first real superstars of the violin, Niccolò Paganini, who died on this day. With his formidable technique, breathtaking virtuosity and futuristic imagination, he pushed and pushed at the boundaries of the violin's technical capabilities, and went on to inspire generations of future fiddlers.

Homesickness
by Emahoy Tsegué-Maryam Guèbrou (1923–2023)

28

Born into one of Ethiopia's wealthiest families, Emahoy Tsegué-Maryam Guèbrou was all set to study at London's prestigious Royal College of Music before she switched course, becoming a nun and remaining largely unknown for decades before word began to emerge of her stunningly distinctive and unusual compositions. This jaunty, rippling, free-flowing, wistful yet cheering piano melody might be as good a cure for homesickness as it's possible to imagine.

Music can be intrinsically linked to memory and evoke strong emotions. What are some of your favourite musical-related memories? What sensations or images come up for you?

African Suite
5: Akinla: Allegro non troppo
by Fela Sowande (1905–1987)

29

Born on this day in Abeokuta, near Lagos, Nigeria, the composer, scholar, ethnomusicologist, educator and organist Fela Sowande is one of the great pioneers of modern African classical music. Written in 1944 and originally broadcast by the BBC, this piece blends West African styles – including the popular dance form highlife and a folk melody from southern Nigeria – with European formalities. Sowande considered it a cornerstone of his argument that West African music could be heard on European terms.

Overture
from *Candide*
by Leonard Bernstein (1918–1990)

30

As a child, I was lucky enough to see *Candide* in London in a concert version in 1989, conducted by Bernstein himself. I was sitting in the front row and was completely transfixed. As he was taking his bow, he turned around and, I'm sure, gave me a wink. Now whenever I hear this, my day is duly winked at; I hope it has the same effect for you.

31

Piano Quintet no. 1 in A minor, op. 30
1: Allegro
by Louise Farrenc (1804–1875)

It probably won't surprise you to learn that women in classical music are generally paid less than their male counterparts. The situation might have been even more iniquitous, though, had it not been for Louise Farrenc, who was born on this day in 1804. As a professor at the Paris Conservatoire, she was paid considerably less than the male professors doing the same job. She fought for a decade to close the gender pay gap and was finally awarded equal pay. A significant milestone for women!

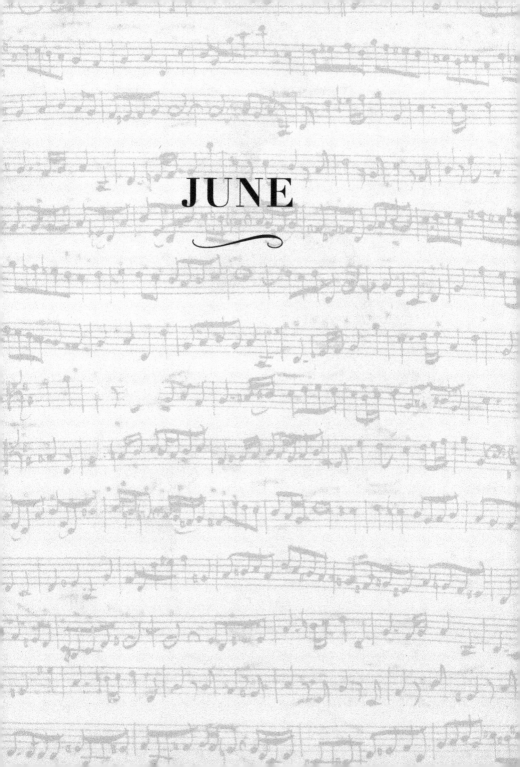

JUNE

Violin Concerto no. 4 in D major, K. 218
2: Andante cantabile
by Wolfgang Amadeus Mozart (1756–1791)

1

Every time I play Mozart myself, I sense a profound sense of kinship with the violin. He gets it to do amazing things – not necessarily the crazy, boundary-pushing pyrotechnics of, say, Paganini (27 May) or von Biber (3 May), although you certainly need a decent technique to play his violin music. But things that feel poetic and lyrical and yearning and human, and are all the more wonderful for it.

Four Choral-Songs, op. 53
1: 'There is Sweet Music'
by Edward Elgar (1857–1934)

2

In this charming 1907 setting of a poem by Alfred, Lord Tennyson, Elgar made a groundbreaking decision to write in two keys simultaneously, with the men singing in G and the women in A flat. It's deceptively difficult to sing, but when a choir gets it right, my goodness it is sweet, sweet music indeed . . .

3

Blumenleben, op. 19
2: 'Veilchen' – 'Violets'
by Dora Pejačević (1885–1923)

Today we hear from a direct contemporary of Elgar, who featured yesterday: a woman breaking her own ground in a very different country and culture. Dora Pejačević is often described as Croatia's first modern symphonist. Although she wrote over a hundred compositions, including dozens of solo piano pieces such as this one, as well as songs, chamber music and orchestral works, very little of her music has been recorded. *Yet*, I have to hope. Yet.

4

Never Saw Him Again
by Mary Lattimore (b.1980)

Harps tend to fall victim to the worst excesses of musical stereotyping, as somehow celestial things, invariably played by beautiful, young, white women with flowing locks and vaguely Pre-Raphaelite features. Pushing five thousand years old, the instrument has long played a role in the music of many diverse cultures, serving everything from mainstream symphony orchestras to avant-garde electronic experiments. Yet I've never heard it like this.

Notice how you feel whilst listening to the harp in Never Saw Him Again *on the opposite page (for example). Think of it as a useful case in point of how things – circumstances, people, events – can surprise us. Think about something or someone who you have been taking somewhat for granted, and try to appreciate them from a fresh perspective.*

5

Ribers no. 8
Traditional Danish, arr. Danish String Quartet

On Danish National Day, some inventive and dynamic musicians with an infectious passion for Nordic folk music. As artists, the Danish String Quartet could not take so-called 'classical music' more seriously, yet they see absolutely no contradiction in building music such as this into their core repertoire. This piece speaks as honestly to who they are as musicians and the rich tradition from which they come as anything else they might care to play.

6

Adagio of Spartacus and Phrygia
from *Spartacus*
by Aram Khachaturian (1903–1978)

The lushest of musical love-letters today from Aram Khachaturian, who was born on this day in 1903. Based on the story of a famous Roman slave revolt, Khachaturian's ballet *Spartacus* contains some of his finest work. This unashamedly romantic episode comes from Act 2, as Spartacus manages to free his lover Phrygia and they are finally reunited. Amid the passionate celebrations, though, listen out for harmonic twists that warn us of the grief to come . . .

Guitar Quintet in D major, G. 448
3. Grave assai – 4. Fandango
by Luigi Boccherini (1743–1805)

7

I love the nocturnal, sensual vibe of this piece, in which a sultry slow movement gives way to an electrifying closing fandango, based on a popular Spanish folk dance. Traditionally, couples with castanets would dance a fandango to a triple-metre guitar accompaniment, and Boccherini captures that tantalizing mood. For all its sizzling vitality, there's a note of longing laced throughout, an energy that keeps it taut and highly charged until the very final bars.

Abendlied – Evening Song
by Robert Schumann (1810–1856)

8

Robert Schumann was born on this day. His was a life marked by intense sorrow and mad grief as well as ecstatic joy, love and beauty. He was a man riven by contradiction and complexity – far too much to sum up within a few minutes of music. And yet – and yet this unbelievably moving song without words for piano, this incandescent 'song of the evening', does somehow distill something of Schumann's spirit. It's three and a half minutes long. I rest my case.

9

Sueño recurrente – Recurring Dream
by Angélica Negrón (b. 1981)

The idiosyncratic Puerto-Rican composer Angélica Negrón writes music for instruments that extend far beyond the traditional classical canon, including accordions, electronics, whistles, toys and robots. She also composes for 'regular' instruments, such as this piece for solo piano. As the title implies, it's a dreamy work; and one that tends to have the effect of lifting me out of wherever I am – conferring an alternative perspective that I am always grateful for.

10

Sleep On: Lullaby
by Mark-Anthony Turnage (b. 1960)

Staying in a world of sleep and dreams, today we say happy birthday to the leading British composer Mark-Anthony Turnage. He wrote this hypnotic suite of lullabies for his young son, but the approach is far from childlike: for all its lyricism and gentle drift, this movement also offers a glimpse into the spiky, dark and often jazz-infused aspects of Turnage's radically distinctive musical style.

How could music help you unwind before bed? Perhaps you can make a plan to introduce more classical music in your daily rituals in order to help you mindfully prepare for rest and reset.

11

Idyll
by Hazel Scott (1920–1981)

Born on this day in Port of Spain, Trinidad and Tobago, Hazel Scott showed such early musical promise that her musician mother took her to New York City at the age of four. By eight, she had won a scholarship to study at the Juilliard School, probably the most iconic classical music conservatoire in the world. Her music, such as this free-form melody, is often improvisatory and infused with the jazz she so adored.

12

Sonatina for piano 4 hands
2: Andante
by György Ligeti (1923–2006)

A little piano music to mark the death on this day of one of the great musical innovators of the twentieth century, who was also capable of transcending the world of avant-garde classical music. This piece, brief as it is, grounds me and brings me a sense of overwhelming calm.

The Salley Gardens
by Benjamin Britten (1913–1976)

13

The quietly moving poem by William Butler Yeats, who was born on this day in 1865, was set by a number of twentieth-century composers. My favourite is this yearningly simple setting by Benjamin Britten, written during World War Two, when he and his partner Peter Pears were on a self-imposed exile to the USA (they were both ardent pacifists).

The Lark Ascending
by Ralph Vaughan Williams (1872–1958)

14

This was written in 1914 but, because of the outbreak of war, only premiered in 1920. It is based on a poem by George Meredith about the song of the skylark, which seemingly effortlessly – although with masterful technical skill – echoes its subject matter through verse. Vaughan Williams' soaring melodic line manages something similarly rhapsodic.

A quick exercise in checking in with yourself: listen to one of the pieces opposite. How does your body respond to the sounds? What sensations do you feel?

Violin sonata no. 3 in C Minor, op. 45
2: Allegretto espressivo alla Romanza
by Edvard Grieg (1843–1907)

15

Violinists are spoiled rotten when it comes to sonata repertoire, and the famous warhorses by the likes of Mozart, Beethoven and Brahms can sometimes get in the way of less obvious gems. But from the very first time I got to play this, having no idea what was in store, I was totally hooked. I hope you will be too.

Mazurka de salon, op. 30
by Teresa Carreño (1853–1917)

16

The mazurka is a sixteenth-century Polish dance form that was brought to popular attention by the great Romantic composer Frédéric Chopin. This one, composed in Paris by a brilliant Venezuelan pianist, conductor, soprano and composer called Teresa Carreño, is a splendid example of how music crosses national lines – and it has the delightful effect of instantly transporting me, in my mind, to some opulent ballroom on the Left Bank, ballgowns ablur and chandeliers aglitter. I love it.

17

Lyric for Strings
by George Walker (1922–2018)

It was this day in 1997 that former Washington, D.C. mayor Marion Barry declared to be 'George Walker Day'. Among many other distinctions, the D.C.-born composer George Walker had become, the previous year, the first African–American to win the Pulitzer Prize for Music. That such a momentous occasion occurred only in 1996 should give us all pause, but still. It's a noteworthy achievement and richly deserved.

18

Violin Sonata in A major
4: Allegretto poco mosso
by César Franck (1822–1890)

Mid-June already, and we are hurtling towards peak wedding season. This glorious violin sonata was written as a wedding present for César Franck's great friend, the violinist Eugène Ysaÿe. It is wistful, yearning, occasionally unbridled in its intensity – and makes the most romantic of musical statements.

Fanfare on Amazing Grace
by Adolphus Hailstork (b. 1941)

19

Today is Juneteenth, or African–American Emancipation Day. Wherever I can, I want to celebrate those incredibly resilient Black composers who have been kept out of the spotlight – or worse – and have overcome. Adolphus Hailstork watched the traumatic news of George Floyd's death in May 2020 – and soon started composing a requiem cantata. Yet, it is a radically positive work: a celebration through music of the victory of our common humanity.

27 Pieces for Viola da Gamba
Prelude
by Carl Friedrich Abel (1723–1787)

20

A two-minute interlude in the key of life, this. It may sound fanciful, but this piece works on me in a way that is instantly physically grounding. From the very first bar I can feel the gently arpeggiated (broken) chords of the viola da gamba start to act on me like some sort of musical gravity, guiding my hunched shoulders down, releasing tension, allowing me to breathe deeper. It's nuts. I don't do regular yoga but I listen to this and I feel that the music is doing something *active* to me.

In the Northern Hemisphere, the days are at their longest this
week, as we reach the Summer Solstice. This is generally a time of
celebration and abundance. Yet in order to grow, we sometimes have
to let go. What's something you need to accept, and let go of,
in order to move forwards?

Porcelain
by Helen Jane Long (b. 1974)

When she's not busy composing music, often for TV shows, adverts and films, the award-winning and versatile British composer Helen Jane Long can be found waterskiing, or perhaps training for the next triathlon, or maybe baking brownies for her colleagues. Not for her the isolated, lofty life of the mind. This refreshing lack of pretension has helped to create music that has proved wildly popular with audiences. If that grates on some classical purists, then the last laugh is surely on her.

Scaramouche for two pianos, op. 165b
3: 'Brazileira' (Mouvement de samba)
by Darius Milhaud (1892–1974)

Darius Milhaud, wrote this little samba on commission from the Scaramouche Theatre Company in Paris, but it was surely influenced by his time spent in Rio de Janeiro between 1917 and 1919. Here he met the composer Heitor Villa-Lobos, who introduced him to local street music. The omnivorously curious Frenchman soaked up all these new sounds and later infused Brazilian-style vibes into much of his music, including this cheeky little caper. Caipirinha optional.

23

The Seasons, op. 37b
6: 'June: Barcarolle'
by Pyotr Ilyich Tchaikovsky (1840–1893)

If yesterday was a day to dream of sipping cachaça-based cocktails on Copacabana beach, today's musical offering serves a somewhat different summer mood. Do you ever get melancholy in June? I know I do. And perhaps Tchaikovsky did too; for me this piece is the quintessence of a certain languid summer restlessness.

24

Six morceaux, op. 85
3: Cavatina
by Joachim Raff (1822–1882)

An unashamedly lovely and romantic little 'morsel' today from a Swiss-German composer who is scarcely spoken of these days, but who in his own time became well known and much admired. Joachim Raff, who died overnight on 24 June, worked at the Hoch Conservatory in Frankfurt, where he employed (praise be!) Clara Schumann and even established a class specifically for female composers – an act of radical early feminism in classical music for which we can all be grateful today.

Argentine Dances, op. 2
2: 'La moza donosa' – 'Dance of the Beautiful Maiden'
by Alberto Ginastera (1916–1983)

25

Today we celebrate one of Argentina's most important composers, Alberto Ginastera, who died on this day. Written in 1937, this is a fantastic example of Ginastera's ability to evoke the vast magnificence of his homeland through music. It's one of those pieces that for me yields something new every time I hear it: whoever that beautiful maiden was, her dance is alluring indeed.

A Lover's Journey
4: 'Shall I Compare Thee to A Summer's Day?'
by Libby Larsen (b. 1950)

26

I hope where you are on this June day it is temperate and lovely, but just in case you're in need of a musical love letter or some sonic sunshine, here's American composer Libby Larsen setting the immortal words of William Shakespeare, Sonnet 18.

27
Bring us, O Lord God
by William Henry Harris (1883–1973)

A dose of divine choral music today from late 1950s England, this is the much-loved choirmaster and organist William Henry Harris setting immortal words by John Donne. It's so beautiful, my advice is simply to try and find three and a half minutes to yourself – and temporarily switch the rest of the world off.

28
Lavender Field
by Karen Tanaka (b. 1961)

Karen Tanaka was born in Tokyo but moved to France in 1986. She has a really eclectic style, but if her work is unified by anything, it's by her love of nature and concern for the environment. Late June is lavender season – in Japan, in France – and hearing this piece at this time of year, I cannot help but imagine vast fields of fragrant, purple flowers. Long may they flourish.

Sometimes there's regeneration in just sitting with your bare, honest feelings. Sit somewhere comfortable, close your eyes, and really listen to the music. Let it wash over you. Do you have any emotional or sensory responses? (Clue: There are no wrong answers!)

29

And I saw a new heaven
by Edgar Bainton (1880–1956)

Edgar Bainton is largely overlooked these days. This anthem, a soaring and glorious mainstay of English church music, is one of the few works that is still performed with any regularity. Yet he was an important figure in what is sometimes described as the English Renaissance, becoming a valiant advocate for contemporary English music, especially in the North of England, where he proved himself an inspiring community leader.

30

1B
by Edgar Meyer (b. 1960)

The multi-award-winning American composer Edgar Meyer writes uncategorizable music that traverses genres such as bluegrass, newgrass and jazz. This mesmerizing track comes from the 2000 Grammy-award-winning album *Appalachian Journey*. If it doesn't transport you somewhere else, instantly and delightfully, perhaps to a sun-drenched, corn-fed American landscape, I'll be amazed!

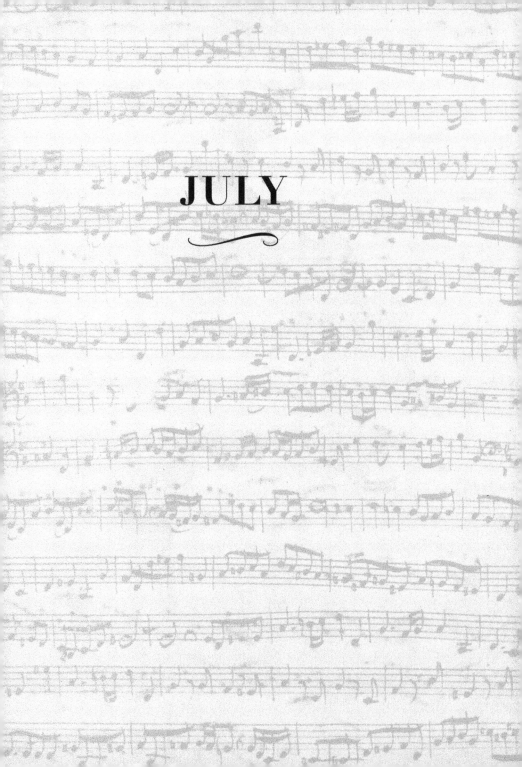

JULY

Avant-dernières pensées – Penultimate Thoughts
3: 'Méditation'
by Erik Satie (1866–1925)

1

A shimmering, startling minute of music to open this new month from Erik Satie, who died on this day.

Trio for piano, violin and cello in D minor
1: Allegro non troppo
by Ethel Smyth (1858–1944)

2

On this day in 1928 the Representation of the People (Equal Franchise) Act became UK law. This landmark in women's rights had been tirelessly campaigned for by the Suffragettes – including today's composer Ethel Smyth, who joined the Women's Social and Political Union in 1910 and, like her friend Mrs Pankhurst, was sent to Holloway Prison.

3

'Glück, das mir verblieb' – Marietta's Lied
from *Die tote Stadt* – *The Dead City*
by Erich Wolfgang Korngold (1897–1957)

This aria from Korngold's smash hit 1920 opera, premiered in Germany when he was just twenty-three, works beautifully in the many different arrangements that have been made of it, but there is something about the sound of the trumpet reaching for Korngold's sustained, yearning notes that I find particularly wrenching.

4

Short Ride in a Fast Machine
by John Adams (b. 1947)

It's the Fourth of July – US Independence Day. I was so spoiled for choice when it came to picking music for today. In the end, amid stiff competition, I decided it was about time we heard from the contemporary master John Adams. His 1986 orchestral fanfare *Short Ride in a Fast Machine* very much does what it says on the tin. In other words, hold on to your hats!

'Kapsberger'
by Giovanni Girolamo Kapsberger (1580–1651)

5

Some cooling, calming, gently repetitious music today from the early Baroque era, and a German–Italian composer. I could listen to music like this all day. If I need a mental reset of the purest sort, it delivers.

Plan & Elevation: The Grounds of Dumbarton Oaks
4: 'The Orangery'
by Caroline Shaw (b. 1982)

6

Caroline Shaw composed this piece while she was the inaugural Music Fellow at Dumbarton Oaks, the historic estate in Georgetown, Washington, D.C. which played host to the famous 1944 conference that led eventually to the foundation of the United Nations. It is a beautiful instance of history, music and architecture converging in one sublime whole.

Although it's often thought of as an elite pursuit, classical music surrounds us. It accompanies many of the films, adverts, historical celebrations and moments that many of us share. Our individual and collective experiences are soundtracked, whether or not we realize it. Can you imagine the world without it? Use this thought exercise to bring mindfulness to your future listening self.

Étude in E major, op. 10 no. 3 ('Tristesse') by Frédéric Chopin (1810–1849)

7

Apparently, Chopin himself thought this was the most beautiful melody he'd ever written. Which is really saying something, because pretty much *every* melody he composed in his tragically short life is a masterpiece. I'm not even kidding. But yes, this one is practically perfect in every way.

Gladiolus Rag by Scott Joplin (c. 1867–1917)

8

I've long had a soft spot for Scott Joplin rags, with their looping sixteen-bar phrases, their teasing melodies, cheekily misbehaving right hands and giddy syncopations. There are so many to choose from you can practically pick a mood, and as July is gladioli season, this one feels particularly appropriate.

9

Cello Concerto in E minor, op. 85
3: Adagio
by Edward Elgar (1857–1934)

Elegiac and fierce and with moments of such blisteringly raw emotion that you emerge from a performance somewhat shredded, this concerto should dispel once and for all the notion of Elgar being an uptight Edwardian who busied himself with a bit of English pastoral here, a spot of nationalist bombast there, and not much else. This concerto has more soul in its little finger than many composers can hope to summon in a lifetime.

10

Song without Words in E major, op. 19 no. 1
by Felix Mendelssohn (1809–1847)

Felix Mendelssohn, born on this day in 1809, perfected the form of a 'song without words', producing eight volumes of the things between 1829 and 1845. What I take from this concept is that, if a piece moves you in a certain way, brings to mind certain images or stories, it doesn't matter if what you're interpreting is what Mendelssohn *intended*. If it gives you what the internet might call many feels, it means what it means.

An American in Paris
by George Gershwin (1898–1937)

11

At seventeen or so minutes, this is one of the longest pieces in the book, but it's also like a mini-universe in musical narrative, so if you can settle in, I promise it will elevate and energize whatever you're up to today. In fact, I'm going to go so far as to say I'm certain there is nothing, no life circumstance, that can't be uplifted by this music.

Trio Sonata in C major, RV 82
2: Larghetto
by Antonio Vivaldi (1678–1741)

12

It's fair to say the mandolin doesn't get a lot of time in the classical solo spotlight. Yet the instrument holds a certain magic. This trio sonata works an absolute treat in the version for the mandolin, especially this spellbinding slow movement, which offers a perfect opportunity for the hushed, expressive eloquence of the mandolin to shine.

13

Another Hike
by Volker Bertlemann, aka Hauschka (b. 1966)

This track, released in 2019, was a chance discovery for me, stumbled upon while I was searching for something else. (Sometimes I really do love the internet.) I'm grateful for that moment of serendipity: this quiet, undulating piece for solo piano from an album celebrating the profound beauty of the natural world has become something to cherish.

14

Les nuits d'été – Summer Nights, op. 7
1: 'Villanelle'
by Hector Berlioz (1803–1869)

For Bastille Day, *la Fête Nationale* in France, we'll hear from one of that country's most forward-thinking, free-spirited and brilliant, if occasionally controversial, composers. I adore this high-spirited, ebullient opening number, which is full of the joys of new love in its first flush.

Just like many of these composers, all humans inevitably experience grief, heartbreak, loneliness and loss at different stages of our lives. Think about the music you tend to turn to in difficult times. What are some of the sonic qualities that you have been most comforted and uplifted by?

15

Virelai (Sus une fontayne)
by Harrison Birtwistle (1934–2022)

Today, we hear from a towering figure in contemporary English music, Sir Harrison Birtwistle, who died in 2022. Prolific and provocative, he was a creator of everything from huge-scale operas and epic orchestral canvases to intimate chamber gems such as this one.

16

Canarios
Traditional improvisation
Version by Jordi Savall (b. 1941)

Here, I give you the 'canario', or canary, a dance craze that spread all over Europe in the late sixteenth and early seventeenth century. The canary is not only referenced in French and Spanish dance manuals of the day, but even has its moment in Shakespeare. To be honest, the canary does sound like a pretty intense move, if the instruction manuals are anything to go by. Maybe don't try this one at home.

Page for Will
by Paul Paccione (b. 1952)

17

This short solo piano piece from 2003, not even two minutes long and dedicated to the composer and music professor Wilbur Ogdon, is a distillation of something that feels very close to beauty for me. It's music that does so much with so little, I feel I hardly need to say more.

Haï luli
by Pauline Viardot (1821–1910)

18

The French–Spanish mezzo-soprano, pedagogue and composer Pauline Viardot was born on this day. Hailing from a ridiculously gifted family, Pauline went on to become an accomplished musician herself, as virtuoso pianist and celebrated opera singer.

19

Three Black Kings
1: 'King of the Magi'
by Duke Ellington (1899–1974)

Right up to his dying day, Duke Ellington championed the cause of Black people through music. *Three Black Kings* was the last thing he wrote, composed on his deathbed in 1974 with the aid of his son. Each movement of the three-parter depicts a Black 'king': Ellington's close friend Martin Luther King, for whom the whole work can be seen as a tribute; King Solomon in the middle; and in this opener, Balthazar, the King of the Magi.

20

Piano Concerto no. 1 in E Minor, op. 11
2: Romance: Larghetto
by Frédéric Chopin (1810–1849)

History was made on this day in 1969 when Neil Armstrong and Buzz Aldrin became the first human beings to walk on the moon. The classical canon is full of musical moonlight – Debussy's *Clair de lune* and Beethoven's Sonata no. 14 spring to mind – but to celebrate that giant leap I wanted to share one of Chopin's piano concertos, laced with longing, which the composer described as '*a sort of meditation . . . by moonlight*'.

Many scientific studies have proved that listening to classical music can help reduce stress and anxiety. Notice how you feel when listening, especially now we are halfway through the year, and make a note of this. See if it changes over the coming months . . .

21

Gottes Zeit ist die allerbeste Zeit – God's time is the best of all times, BWV 106
by Johann Sebastian Bach (1685–1750)
and György Kurtág (b. 1926)

Today, a work of pure musical serenity that engenders in me an inner state of peace, even resolution. I am reminded every time I hear it of the quiet but undeniable miracle that music can do this.

22

Italian Dance
by Madeleine Dring (1923–1977)

A quick shot of musical sunshine today, courtesy of this ebullient little dance for oboe by the British composer, actress, lyricist, cabaret performer and cartoonist Madeleine Dring. She was very much her own woman, and in her classical compositions she forged her own musical voice. It's a charming one, I hope you agree.

Pieces for clavecin: Book 3, 14th order
'Le Rossignol-en-amour' – 'The Nightingale in Love'
by François Couperin (1668–1733)

23

First of all, I love the idea of a nightingale in love: what an image. And from the moment I encountered it I fell hard for this music by Couperin 'the great', as the famous French Baroque harpsichordist was known in his time. In his graceful modalities, dance-like rhythms and the agility he demands from a player, you can almost hear a sonic path being laid that will lead to the future of so much keyboard music.

Faire is the Heaven
by William Henry Harris (1883–1973)

24

Composed in 1925, this glorious five-minute anthem by the largely neglected English composer William Henry Harris sets a verse from 'An Hymne of Heavenly Beautie' by the great Renaissance poet Edmund Spenser (c. 1552–1599). It's so beautiful, I think I'll leave it there.

25

Particles
by Ólafur Arnalds (b. 1986)

Something odd happened to me when I first heard this. I had an involuntary response: I wept. I can't tell you why I was so profoundly moved, physiologically as well as emotionally; I guess it's all part of the mystery and miracle of music, why certain combinations of notes and rhythms work on us, enchant us, in the way they do.

26

Déploration sur la mort de Jehan Ockeghem
by Josquin des Prez (c. 1450–1521)

The composer Josquin des Prez reached a greater level of fame than probably any musician before him because of his enthusiastic embrace of modern technology – in this case the newly invented printing press. Many of his masses were printed in his lifetime, picking up admirers including the seminal Reformation theologian Martin Luther.

Piano Trio in G minor, op. 17
3: Andante
by Clara Schumann (1819–1896)

27

It's high summer, July 1846. Robert Schumann and his wife Clara travel to Norderney, an island off the North Sea coast of Germany, in a bid to try and help Schumann's mental health. While there, Clara suffers a miscarriage and at some point around this time she composes this astonishingly wonderful music. How she manages it, I cannot imagine. It's beautiful beyond belief, and my heart breaks for all that she is going through.

Partita no. 2 in D Minor, BWV 1004
5: Chaconne
by Johann Sebastian Bach (1685–1750)

28

Today, on the anniversary of Bach's death, time to hear the 'Bach Chaconne'. Many composers consider it the gold standard, the ultimate musical benchmark.

This is everything.

What do you picture when you listen to – for example –
Hallelujah Junction on the next page? Why not close your eyes and
think about it. Then consider trying to create a different piece of art
altogether. A sketch? A painting? A dance? Just for you.

Hallelujah Junction
1st movement
by John Adams (b. 1947)

29

This piece has one of the most thrilling openings of any piece ever written. *Hallelujah*, indeed!

Lo, the full, final sacrifice, op. 26
by Gerald Finzi (1901–1956)

30

This work moves from brooding interiority in the opening bars into the most expansive, glorious, rapturously life-affirming and moving 'Amen' I may have ever heard.

31

En rêve, nocturne
by Franz Liszt (1811–1886)

The spectacle of young women shrieking, sobbing and swooning at the sight of their musical idols might seem a relatively modern phenomenon. But before there were Elvis fanatics, Beatlemania, Swifties and BTS' ARMY there was so-called 'Lisztomania'. Liszt, a Hungarian pianist, composer and pedagogue, overcame poverty to become music's first real, bona fide 'celebrity'. I've chosen a piece he wrote in old age: a contemplative and poignant nocturne.

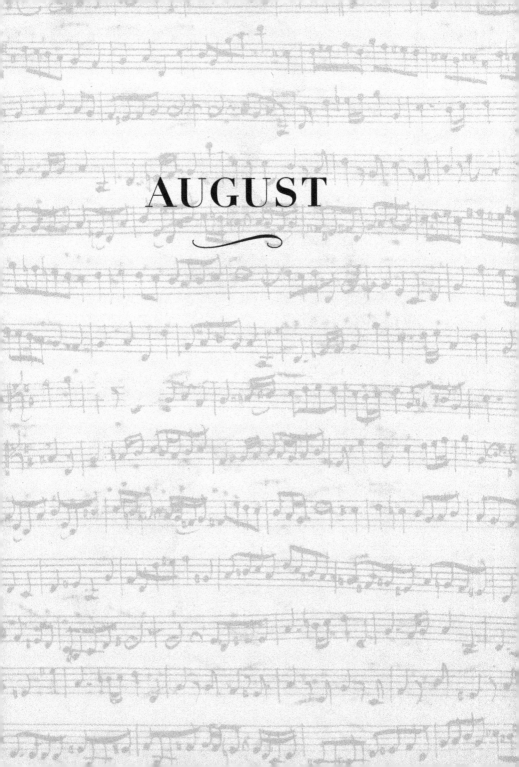

AUGUST

Trauer – Sorrow
1: 'Vasara' – 'Summer'
by Pēteris Vasks (b. 1946)

The Latvian landscape, folklore and culture are central to the composer Pēteris Vasks' writing, and especially in his choral works. In this sublime 1978 meditation on summer in his homeland, for women's choir, he combines a modernist, contemporary sensibility with a deep reverence for ancient singing traditions. The effect is a shimmering, multi-faceted jewel.

Let us go, then, duly soul-nourished, into this new month . . .

To be Sung of a Summer Night on the Water
1: Slow but not dragging
by Frederick Delius (1862–1934)

This dreamy, textless choral idyll, written during the Great War but only premiered in 1920, conjures a particularly heady atmosphere. I find it the perfect soundtrack to a summer night.

3

Children's Suite
2: 'Cheerful Walk'
by Galina Ustvolskaya (1919–2006)

Daughter of a lawyer and schoolteacher, Galina Ustvolskaya, who came of age in the first generation after the Russian Revolution of 1917, was hardly destined for a career in classical music. But she beat the odds and went on to become one of the very few Soviet women composers – in fact, Soviet women musicians of any kind – to gain prominence on the international scene.

4

Azul
3: 'Transit'
by Osvaldo Golijov (b. 1960)

Premiered by the great cellist Yo-Yo Ma and Brooklyn-based ensemble The Knights on this day in 2006, this contemplative, rhythmically surprising and truly unusual cello concerto by the Argentine composer Osvaldo Golijov takes the Spanish word for 'blue' as its title. I picture a vast ocean of possibility; it's fair to say Golijov dives right in.

How have you been feeling after listening to this week's pieces?
Notice any responses in your body. Do you feel comfortable or
uncomfortable? Do you feel an emotional reaction or
a sensory reaction? Both?

5

Clarinet Sonata in E flat major, op. 167
1: Allegretto
by Camille Saint-Saëns (1835–1921)

With woodwind instruments drastically less well served for solo repertoire than their stringed counterparts, Saint-Saëns took it upon himself in the last year of his existence to contribute one sonata apiece for oboe, clarinet, bassoon, flute and cors anglais. With minimal fuss, here he gives the clarinet a powerful calling card and takes the instrument forward into the twentieth century. It's a gem.

6

Ride Through
by Eleanor Alberga (b. 1949)

On Jamaica Independence Day, music from one of that country's most magnificent musical daughters. Born in Kingston, Alberga was just five when she decided she wanted to be a pianist. Later she came to the UK to study at the Royal Academy of Music, and her work as a composer has been heard everywhere from the soundtrack of *Snow White and the Seven Dwarves* to classical music's biggest knees-up, The Last Night of the Proms.

Dum transisset Sabbatum 1
by John Taverner (c. 1490–1545)

7

A moment of sonic respite and repose today. If modern life is getting you down, if it's all a bit much, as it often is for me, I would urge you to try and take a moment, close your eyes, and press play on this glowing rapturous, centuries-old sacred motet which is barely even ten minutes long but somehow remakes the world.

Rêve d'enfant – Dream of a Child, op. 14
by Eugène Ysaÿe (1858–1931)

8

Perhaps it's being a mother of little ones myself, but there is something that always hits me hard when I learn about composers writing music for their children. Here is a serene and lyrical lullaby, composed in 1894 while the great Belgian violinist and composer Eugène Ysaÿe was on a long concert tour. He dedicated it to his youngest son, Antoine. Bless.

9

Mattinata – Morning
by Ruggero Leoncavallo (1857–1919)

In 1904, this music was the first piece ever to be written espe-cially for the Gramophone and Typewriter Company, recorded by legendary tenor Enrico Caruso with the composer himself on the piano. Leoncavallo, who died on this day, produced many songs and operas throughout his career, but apart from this historic number, he is otherwise only really known for his one-act verismo opera *Pagliacci* ('Clowns', 1892).

10

Studies for Player Piano
Study no. 6
by Conlon Nancarrow (1912–1997)

Music today from the fascinating Conlon Nancarrow, an avant-garde American-born composer who later became a Mexican citizen. A Communist who fought in the Spanish Civil War, joining the Abraham Lincoln Brigade to defend the Spanish Republic against General Franco, Nancarrow was extremely reclusive and barely known outside of his own circle until the 1980s. But at that point, a certain fascination with his music started to grow among a sector of contemporary music lovers and fellow composers.

Locus iste
by Anton Bruckner (1824–1896)

11

It was on this day in 1869 that the late Romantic Austrian composer Anton Bruckner composed this astonishingly beautiful motet for four unaccompanied voice parts (soprano, alto, tenor, bass). This three-minute motet makes a strong case for the argument that there is little more powerful in music – or indeed, in life – than the sound of intertwining human voices.

Nyári este – Summer Evening
by Zoltán Kodály (1882–1967)

12

This spacious, light-filled orchestral work, written in 1906 by the Hungarian composer Zoltán Kodály, is one of the longest pieces I've included. It lasts almost eighteen minutes, which is a good amount of time, I find, in which to let it open up and expand across a pleasant evening activity – sitting with a glass of wine, preparing dinner al fresco, taking a walk in the last embers of the day's warmth (hopefully).

Remember a time when music helped to lift your mood and soothe your soul. Perhaps it was a concert with friends or loved ones; or perhaps you were listening to music in your room or on a walk or journey? Do you think journalling about those moments might help you glean some general insights about yourself?

The Darkness is No Darkness
by Judith Bingham (b. 1952)

13

Here, British composer Judith Bingham sets text from Psalm 139
... I'll say no more: see you tomorrow.

Thou wilt keep him in perfect peace
by Samuel Sebastian Wesley (1810–1876)

14

Born, illegitimate, in London on this day, Samuel Sebastian Wesley
supposedly got his middle name because of his composer father's
obsession with Johann Sebastian Bach. (I get this. My youngest
son's name is Joe.) This anthem is, to me, a particularly majestic
example of Wesley's talents, delivering four blissful minutes of, yes,
perfect choral peace.

15

Sospiri, op. 70
by Edward Elgar (1857–1934)

I think about the first performance of this piece, which took place at the Queen's Hall in London on this day in 1914, and it seems to freeze a moment in time. Who knows what was in Elgar's head and heart at the time of putting pen to manuscript paper? But as a listener, knowing what was to lie around the corner, it is hard not to hear in the wrenching musical upheavals that disrupt its mood of serene pastoral the very essence of a farewell.

16

Partita no. 3 in E major, BWV 1006
1: Prelude
by Johann Sebastian Bach (1685–1750)

This piece for solo violin always works on me like a shot of musical caffeine. (Bach did, as it happens, write a Coffee Cantata but that's for another year.) In just a hundred seconds or so this piece has the effect of apparently rearranging the molecules around me, making me see and think more clearly. (I know! Sounds crazy. But: true. And cheaper than an espresso . . .)

The Wife
by Jocelyn Pook (b. 1960)

17

Jocelyn Pook is an award-winning British composer and former violist and pianist who first came to prominence when she started collaborating with film-maker Stanley Kubrick. Pook writes for opera, concert hall, stage and particularly screen; hers is a musical sensibility, rich in narrative eloquence, that seems particularly well placed to tell powerful stories. This soothing yet unsettling track, for example, comes from the score to *The Wife*, a 2017 film staring Glenn Close and Jonathan Pryce.

Memories in Watercolour, op. 1
4: 'Blue'
by Tan Dun (b. 1957)

Happy birthday to the Chinese composer Tan Dun, writer of such memorable film scores as Ang Lee's *Crouching Tiger, Hidden Dragon* (2000) and winner of multiple awards, including an Oscar, a Grammy and a BAFTA. Dun's music often draws upon organic materials, including rock and water. Although not explicit, I can definitely hear something of that sensibility in this delicate, shimmering piano piece.

One of the most wonderful things about discovering new music is the ability to share it with others. Perhaps jot down a new playlist or the names of any newly discovered composers and their backlists that you plan to explore or introduce to friends.

Hora Unirii
by George Enescu (1881–1955)

19

I first encountered this effervescent folk-style dance thanks to the visionary violinist Daniel Hope, who was putting a tribute album together for Yehudi Menuhin, one of the greatest violinists of all time. Menuhin had been profoundly shaped by his collaborations with Enescu, a Romanian violinist, pianist, composer and conductor, whom Menuhin believed was the greatest all-round musician of the twentieth century. This piece is certainly like an energy shot in the arm, not even two minutes of Romanian gypsy glory.

Piano Concerto no. 2 in C minor, op. 18
2: Adagio sostenuto
by Sergei Rachmaninov (1873–1943)

20

This is the sort of unashamedly wonderful piece that some classical music critics pride themselves on deriding – for being, I don't know, 'cheesy' or 'populist'. Whatever. (As far as I'm concerned, this is precisely why 'Classical Music' has such an image problem.) To these people I say: relax, guys! It's okay to get off on this music even though *everyone else in the rest of the world does too*! Being universally loved does not detract from the concerto's genius. Quite the opposite.

21

G-Spot Tornado
by Frank Zappa (1940–1993)

I'll never forget being at the BBC *Proms* one night in the summer of 2013 and feeling as though the Royal Albert Hall might just lift off, such was the zany and flamboyant exuberance of this work by the experimental American musician, filmmaker and activist Frank Zappa.

22

'La fleur que tu m'avais jetée' – 'The flower that you threw to me'
from *Carmen*
by Georges Bizet (1838–1875)

Georges Bizet suffered from crushing disappointment and lack of critical appreciation in his all too brief life. His thirtieth (!) attempt at an opera, *Carmen*, was a spectacular failure at its premiere, which took place just three months before he died.

This sensational aria from Act 2 is my favourite moment in the whole opera. It's one of the most splendid love songs, but naturally, this *being* opera, it won't be long before it all ends in tears . . .

Disco-Toccata
by Guillaume Connesson (b. 1970)

23

Today's composer is one of the bright lights on France's contemporary scene; he has also been Composer-in-Residence at the Royal Scottish National Orchestra. Connesson had me at the title *Disco-Toccata*, but I subsequently fell in love with the energy and vitality of his music.

Four Pieces, op. 78
2: Romance
by Jean Sibelius (1865–1957)

24

I have a real weakness for gorgeous romantic instrumental chamber works such as this one. I know it's a little basic, but I always find the sheer simplicity of two melodic lines combining in a way that is so much greater than the sum of their parts quietly magical; it gets me every time.

25

Chroma: Transit of Venus
by Joby Talbot (b. 1971)

It was ballet that first introduced me, inadvertently, to Talbot's music, via his 2006 collaboration with leading choreographer Wayne McGregor on *Chroma*, the multi-award-winning one-act work from which this comes. I remember going to see the ballet, and being utterly transfixed: it was one of those rare experiences that I knew would stay imprinted on my mind for ever.

26

Set Me as a Seal
by Nico Muhly (b. 1981)

This early choral piece sets words from the Old Testament text *Song of Solomon*, also known as the *Song of Songs*, whose sensuous, mysterious, at times even ecstatic language has inspired composers through the ages, including Nico Muhly, who was born on this day.

Note your three favourite classical composers and genres.
Have these changed as the year has progressed?

27

'Deep River'
from *24 Negro Melodies*, op. 59 no. 10
by Samuel Coleridge-Taylor (1875–1912)

We've met a few classical composers this year who sought to reflect their heritage through music. Born in London to a Sierra Leonean father and English mother, Samuel Coleridge-Taylor (whom Edward Elgar once described as *'far and away the cleverest'* of the new generation of composers) placed himself firmly in this tradition.

28

'Sleep'
from *Five Elizabethan Songs*
by Ivor Gurney (1890–1937)
arr. Iain Farrington (b. 1977)

I find this piece, especially in this stunning arrangement for tenor and string orchestra, desperately moving. It haunts me – but in the very best possible way that wonderful art and human stories can.

Idyll
5: Adagio
by Leoš Janáček (1854–1928)

29

The *Idyll*, for string orchestra, is only the second large-scale orchestral work of Janáček's that survives. Completed on this day in 1878, it had its premiere later that year, conducted by the composer himself, and must have felt like a momentous occasion: his hero Anton Dvořák, whose influence can be strongly felt and heard throughout the piece, was in the audience.

The Seasons
4: 'Summer'
by Thea Musgrave (b. 1928)

30

As we head towards the close of summer, in the northern hemisphere at least, a last nod to the season today from one of the most formidable and prolific British composers of our time, the Scottish-born, New York-dwelling Thea Musgrave.

31

Ich wandle unter Blumen – I wander among flowers
by Alma Mahler (1879–1964)

An intriguing sliver of a song to end the month from the ever-enigmatic Alma Mahler, Gustav Mahler's wife, who was born on this day. Although Alma had been crazy about composing in her early years, she left behind only seventeen songs at the end of her turbulent and chequered life, giving us only the merest hint of the talent that might have been.

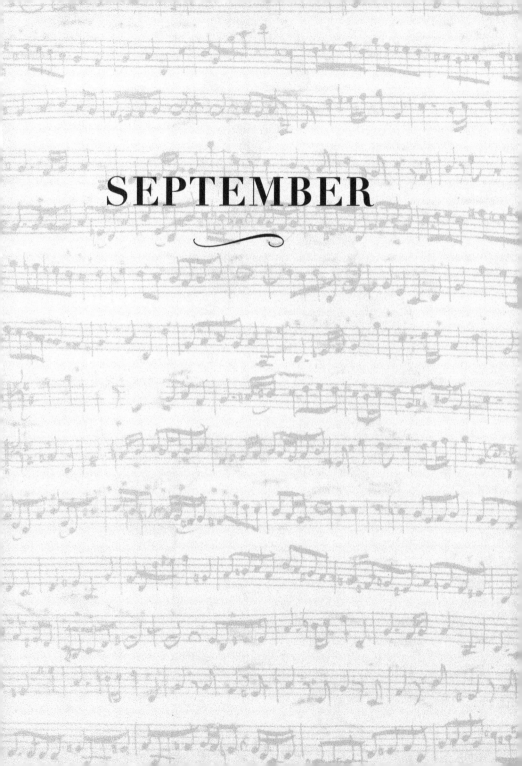

SEPTEMBER

'September'
from *Vier letzte Lieder – Four Last Songs*
by Richard Strauss (1864–1949)

1

And just like that: September has come. Strauss was in the very autumn of his life, eighty-four years old, when he composed his *Four Last Songs*. They were never published or performed in his lifetime – he died the following year – but hold iconic status among singers. As a legacy, there's nothing else quite like them. *Four Last Songs* look not back but forward, to death, yet they do so with tremendous peacefulness and serenity. I honestly think it's one of the most beautiful things I've ever heard.

Umbrian Scene
by Ulysses Kay (1917–1995)

2

I love this piece. I mean, *I love it*. I love the chromatic colours, the unusual tonal palette. I love its timelessness. I love the lyrical, rich harmonies of his orchestration: at times, the romantic lushness; at others, the almost polyphonic sparseness. I love the sense of space and yet drama and something that all great music has: an ineffable quality, of just being *it*.

3

'The Flight of the Bumblebee'
from *The Tale of Tsar Sultan*
by Nikolai Rimsky-Korsakov (1844–1908)

In the opera, this music takes place at the end of a tableau scene in Act 3, during which the magical Swan-Bird has transformed the Tsar's son into a bumblebee, so that he can fly away to his father, who does not know that he's alive. It is characteristic of Rimsky-Korsakov, one of the most brilliant orchestrators in musical history, that he is able to evoke this breakneck flight in a flurry of notes.

4

'Bella figlia dell'amore' – 'Beautiful daughter of love'
from *Rigoletto*
by Giuseppe Verdi (1813–1901)

It seems inconceivable now, given the marginalization of opera and classical music in our own society, but back in the day composers such as Verdi were the pop stars of their time.

This piece is as brilliant as it is beautiful: a complex and intricate confection that in Verdi's hands comes across as apparently effortless.

Take yourself to a garden or park and listen to 'The Flight of the Bumblebee' (opposite). Then note down all the sounds you can hear. Do you think the way you are hearing it might be different in another context?

5

Clarinet Quintet in A major, K. 581
2: Larghetto
by Wolfgang Amadeus Mozart (1756–1791)

Exemplifying ideals of friendship and human connections throughout, this piece combines Mozart's inestimable gifts, somehow taking the best of his opera, his chamber music and his instrumental concertos and weaving them into something whose emotional impact feels disproportionate to what it is: a few pages of manuscript paper, covered in dots of ink, written in a hurry.

6

Elegy in D flat major, op. 17
by Alexander Glazunov (1865–1936)

As a musically inclined teenager in St. Petersburg, Alexander Glazunov studied with the leading composer of the day, Rimsky-Korsakov, who we met earlier this month (3 September). Glazunov went on to become a significant figure in Russian music. As well as taking on the directorship of the St Petersburg Conservatoire, he produced symphonies, ballets, instrumental concertos and smaller-scale works such as this lyrical *Elegy* for cello and piano. Lush and unashamedly romantic, it wears its gigantic heart on its sleeve.

12 Sonatas, op. 16
3: Sonata terza
by Isabella Leonarda (1620–1704)

7

It was on this day in Novara, Italy, that a remarkable figure in the history of Western music was born: a woman named Isabella Leonarda, who managed to produce at least two hundred compositions in her lifetime while she lived as a nun at the Collegio di Sant'Orsola. Full of bold harmonies, improvisatory passages that call for great virtuosity, and moments of real grace, it's no wonder Leonarda reportedly became known as the '*Muse of Novara*'.

Fragile N.4
by Dustin O'Halloran (b. 1971)

8

Recording of the 2010 album, *Lumiere*, from whence this piece comes, took place in an ancient church in Berlin, a rustic Italian farmhouse and an old New York bookshop. It was during this process that O'Halloran apparently discovered he could hear music as colours, a neurological phenomenon known as 'synesthesia'.

Do you see, or even hear, any colours when listening to music?
What about images? Are they abstract or conceptual?
Take a moment to really listen and note down with curiosity
what you experience.

Che si può fare – What am I to do?
by Barbara Strozzi (1619–1677)

9

This haunting song is written on a passacaglia (variations over a bass line) that consists of the first four notes of a descending D minor scale. As it happens, it's a bass line that crops up again and again in twentieth-century jazz and blues (for example 'Hit the road Jack').

Come, ye sons of Art, away (Birthday Ode for Queen Mary)
5: 'Strike the viol'
by Henry Purcell (1659–1695)
arr. Christina Pluhar (b. 1965)

10

Henry Purcell's original piece, written to celebrate Queen Mary II's birthday in 1694, is sparkling enough, but I love what Pluhar does here, bringing the freshness and wit of her musical imagination to an already vigorous and at times ecstatic score, which praises, above all, the joys of music.

11

'In Paradisum'
from *Trinity Requiem*
by Robert Moran (b. 1937)

The chapel of St Paul at Trinity Church, Wall Street, sits across the street from the former World Trade Center in downtown Manhattan. Following the terror attacks of 11 September 2001, the chapel became a hub and a haven for people. In 2011, to commemorate the tenth anniversary of the attacks, American composer Robert Moran was commissioned to write a Requiem for Trinity Church's Youth Chorus. He opted for simplicity, setting the sweet, pure voices of children against an accompaniment of cellos, organ and harp.

12

Adagio and Allegro for cello and piano, op. 70
by Robert Schumann (1810–1856)

On Robert and Clara Schumann's wedding anniversary (they married on this day in 1840), we'll hear Schumann in full-on love-song mode. It is simply a joy to hear him writing from such a place of unalloyed happiness.

'Nachtwandler' – 'Sleepwalker'
from *Cabaret Songs*
by Arnold Schoenberg (1874–1951)

13

Arnold Schoenberg was born on this day – and with that fateful occurrence, the path of classical music changed for ever. Bam. Schoenberg is one of those composers – along with the likes of Monteverdi, Bach, Liszt, Beethoven and Wagner – who represent a metaphorical fork in the musical road after which nothing is ever quite the same again. As a composer working in his wake, you can choose to emulate Schoenberg or reject Schoenberg but you sure as hell cannot *ignore* Schoenberg.

Berceuse, P. 38
by Ottorino Respighi (1879–1936)

14

Today we're back to the lushly orchestrated sound world of the Romantic era. This early piece for string orchestra, written when Ottorino Respighi was only in his early twenties, caught me off-guard the first time I heard it and I fell for it hard.

Consider the songs or pieces of music you loved growing up.
Do you still listen to them now? Do you think you have changed?
Do you think the music has changed? Might the music have
changed you? Or is it just a matter of perspective?

Piano Quintet no. 2 in E major, op. 31
1: Andante sostenuto – Allegro grazioso
by Louise Farrenc (1804–1875)

15

An absolute cracker of a piano quintet today from Louise Farrenc. Despite her impressive achievements, she slipped, like so many musical women throughout history, into relative oblivion. This piece, for example, went out of print for decades and was only recorded in the 1990s, well over a century after her death. It more than deserves its place in the golden canon of nineteenth-century chamber music.

Danzón no. 2
by Arturo Márquez (b. 1950)

16

Although the *danzón* as a dance form has its origins in eighteenth-century Europe and was refined in nineteenth-century Cuba, it has become synonymous with parts of Mexico. And so, on Mexico's Independence Day, let us jump on this magic sonic carpet and be conveyed back to the 1940s and the golden age of the *danzón*.

17

Schulwerk – Music for Children
'Gassenhauer nach Hans Neusiedler (1536)'
by Carl Orff (1895–1982)

I first came across this when the Oscar-winning film-maker Sam Mendes revealed to me that it was *this* piece of European classical music, unlikely as it sounds, that helped him find a distinctive sound world for his American-suburbia-set masterpiece of a first movie, the multi-award-winning *American Beauty*, which came out on this day in 1999.

18

Ciaccona
by Francesca Caccini (1587–1641)

Born in Florence on this day, the early Baroque composer Francesca Caccini is thought to be the first woman ever to write an opera. Well-educated and accomplished, also as a singer, lutenist and poet, Caccini was described as *'always gracious and generous'* and a woman of refinement and wit. I think those qualities are evident in her music. Today, we'll hear her take on the chaconne, or *'ciaccona'*, which was one of the hottest dance forms of the day. It's a real foot-tapper.

Ave Maria 1
by Rihards Dubra (b. 1964)

19

A luminous and calming choral interlude today from the contemporary Latvian composer Rihards Dubra, this setting of the
thirteenth-century anonymous Ave Maria text was written in 1989,
shortly before the end of the Soviet occupation of Dubra's homeland.

Violin Concerto in D minor, op. 47
2: Adagio di molto
by Jean Sibelius (1865–1957)

20

If you're only going to write one concerto in life, it may as well be
this one.

My mum has always loved this concerto and she would often
stick it on at home. Even as a child it spoke to me profoundly; one
of my 'before-and-after' pieces. The second movement in particular
is extraordinary: a mercilessly beautiful, eight-minute benediction.

The Autumn Equinox is a time to mark the change of the seasons.
You might turn slightly inwards, as the nights start to get darker.
Now is a time for gratitude and preparation for the coming months.
Celebrate five things you appreciate and value right now, and
consider how you might make space for many more . . .

Autumn Crocus
by Billy Mayerl (1902–1959)

21

As a composer, Billy Mayerl produced over three hundred piano pieces. Usually classed as 'light music' (which does a disservice to his considerable inventiveness), many of them were named after trees and flowers, such as today's charming autumnal crocus.

'Entry of the Gods into Valhalla'
from *Das Rheingold*
by Richard Wagner (1813–1883)

22

As a man, Richard Wagner seems to have been pretty vile, full of unspeakable ideology. (Hitler was a fan.) And yet, perplexingly, his music is often touched with the divine, and powerful, and among the most influential there has ever been.

23

Prendi per me sei libero – Take it,
because of me you are free
by Maria Malibran (1808–1836)

Before there was Maria *Callas*, there was Maria *Malibran*, the original diva and operatic superstar. This aria was written by Malibran herself when she sang the role of Adina in Donizetti's opera *L'elisir d'amore*. For such a short life, her legacy is remarkable.

24

Across the Stars (Love Theme from Star Wars Episode II:
Attack of the Clones)
by John Williams (b. 1932)

Lest anyone raise an eyebrow about the inclusion of *Star Wars* in a compendium of classical music, I'm just going to state that John Williams is simply one of the greatest composers of the past century, end of story. Magnificent!

Les Boréades
Act 4, scene 4: Entry of the muses, zephyrs, seasons, hours and arts
by Jean-Philippe Rameau (1683–1764)

25

Jean-Philippe Rameau was fifty when his first opera was produced and *Les Boréades* (1763) was his last. It was never produced in Rameau's lifetime and wasn't staged properly until the late twentieth century, despite containing some fabulous music – including this dreamy orchestral interlude from Act 4.

Du bist die Ruh – You are peace, D. 776
by Franz Schubert (1797–1828)

26

Schubert, who died from syphilis at the age of thirty-one, never married or had a long-term relationship. This rapturous hymn to enduring love offers a glimpse into the heart of a highly emotional human who would surely have aspired to a lasting romantic union had he not been wrenched from the world by such a cruel disease.

Listen to a piece from this week. Try to connect it with a natural landscape you have visited. Do you picture a lake, a mountain, a forest? Or perhaps somewhere else entirely . . . What does the natural world mean to you?

In manus tuas
by John Sheppard (c. 1515–1558)

27

Today we will journey back through the centuries for a spot of sumptuous Renaissance polyphony from the English composer John Sheppard. Sheppard gets a lot less airtime than his more famous contemporaries, possibly because so much of his output has been lost. If this four minutes of music is anything to go by, that represents an unbearable loss. But at least there's this; there's this.

Overture
from *The Bartered Bride*
by Bedřich Smetana (1824–1884)

28

One to blast away the cobwebs today. Consider this a six-ish-minute energy shot courtesy of Bedřich Smetana, who was one of the great founding fathers of Czech classical music.

29
Un Regalo – A Gift
by Mark Simpson (b. 1988)

Mark Simpson is nothing if not thoughtful. A visceral, virtuosic composer who is also an outstanding clarinettist with a major solo career, the young Liverpudlian has been lighting up the classical music scene since 2006. He is also an ardent advocate for the benefits of music education and opening up a world that can be hideously elitist.

30
'Au fond du temple saint' – 'At the back of the holy temple'
from *The Pearl Fishers*
by Georges Bizet (1838–1875)

I was listening to this on the tube and a fellow passenger actually touched me on the arm and asked if I was okay. 'Yes!' I gasped, 'I'm fine!' but in truth I was practically expiring due to the beauty of this piece of music. We're talking *crazy-beautiful*. Seriously. I don't know how anyone could possibly listen to it impassively: it's insane.

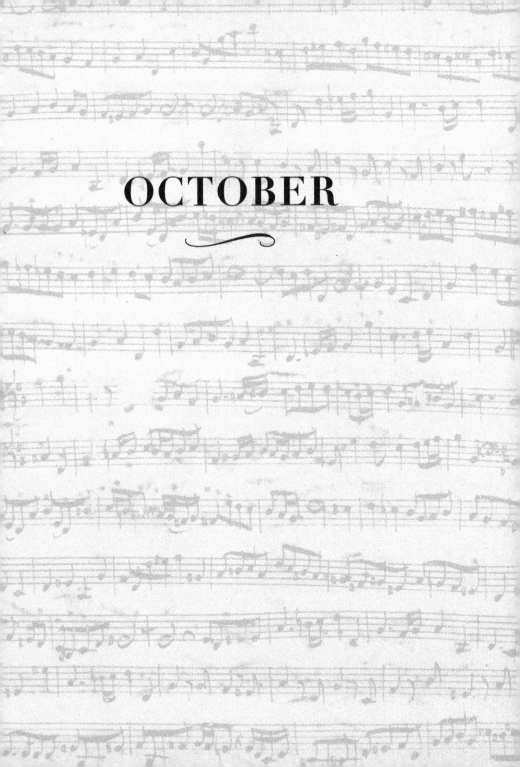

OCTOBER

A Downland Suite
3: Minuet
by John Ireland (1879–1962)

1

John Ireland is sometimes described as an English 'impressionist' and this work can be read as a kind of musical love-letter to the English landscape, about which he was passionate. Also, fact: there's nothing like the sound of a good brass band, and this, in my opinion, is an ideal piece to show that sound off in all its glory.

Kol nidrei, op. 47
by Max Bruch (1838–1920)

2

The *Kol nidrei,* sung on the eve of Yom Kippur, is a mournful, ancient synagogue chant which in Aramaic means 'all vows'. Bruch would likely have encountered its affecting melody through the cantor-in-chief of Berlin, Abraham Jacob Lichtenstein, who actively encouraged his interest in Jewish folk songs.

3

Music for 18 Musicians
'Pulses'
by Steve Reich (b. 1936)

I will never, ever, forget the first time I heard this, and the immediate, life-changing, mind-altering thrill it gave me. Even today, many years after my first time, *Music for 18 Musicians* has lost none of its power: I find it beautiful and reverberant, mathematically precise yet somehow organic, warm, life-giving, oxygenating, pulsating, magical.

4

Melodia en La menor [Canto de Octubre]
by Astor Piazzolla (1921–1992)

In its blend of classical music, jazz and old Buenos Aires street tango, this piece is a fine example of the 'nueva tango' style that Piazzolla – who had always been omnivorously curious about other types of music – pioneered. This is an excellent piece, I find, to enjoy on an autumnal evening.

Autumn Gardens
3: Giocoso e leggiero
by Einojuhani Rautavaara (1928–2016)

5

This piece, written in 1999, towards the end of the Finnish composer Einojuhani Rautavaara's life, is a good example of the way he fore-grounds a mystical and evocative atmosphere over other potential considerations. Music, for obvious reasons of structure and form, is often compared to architecture, but Rautavaara finds a garden to be the more appropriate metaphor for his work.

If the silver bird could speak
by Eleanor Alberga (b. 1949)

6

Despite the intersectional odds stacked against a Black woman of her generation making her way in this industry, the redoubtable Eleanor Alberga has never let either race or gender stand in her way. Alberga was born and raised in Kingston, Jamaica and moved to London in 1970. Her vivid, candid music, which includes orchestral, vocal and chamber music as well as opera, is a distinctive blend of both sides of her heritage.

In our busy modern lives, sometimes we can take the turning of the seasons for granted. Try to notice all the autumnal things you encounter today. Maybe you can collect a particularly beautiful fallen leaf and place it between the pages of this book, as a physical reminder of this moment to come back to.

Hear Us
by Anna Thorvaldsdóttir (b. 1977)

7

Today we hear an ancient Icelandic hymn, or prayer, given a sublime modern treatment. I don't really want to say more, only to give you space to receive this music, wherever you are at.

But, my gosh, what a simple, and powerful, human entreaty: *hear us*. Hear us.

Canzoni overo sonate concertate per chiesa e camera,
a 2–3, libro terzo, op. 12
20: Ciaccona
by Tarquinio Merula (c. 1595–1665)

8

Not a name we hear too often these days, the Italian composer Tarquinio Merula was nevertheless a notable musical figure in the early Baroque period. Cosmopolitan in outlook and progressive in style, Merula played a key role in the development of many musical forms and innovations that are still in use across multiple musical genres today.

9

Ave maris stella
by Cecilia McDowall (b. 1951)

As this exquisite and moving 2008 setting of the *Ave maris stella* shows, Cecilia McDowall – who came late to composing, in her forties – has gone on to become a distinctive musical voice, winning, in 2014, the prestigious British Composer Award for choral writing. I love her story and hope it might provide hope and inspiration for anyone who still dreams of pursuing a creative path, whoever they are and whatever stage they are at in life.

10

Suite for violin and piano
21: 'Mother and Child'
by William Grant Still (1895–1978)

For this three-part suite, composed in 1943, William Still took as his inspiration works of 1930s visual art associated with the cultural movement known as the Harlem Renaissance, that tremendous social and artistic flowering that emerged out of the Black mecca of Harlem between the 1910s and 1930s.

Symphony no. 9 in D minor
3: Adagio: Langsam, feierlich – slowly, solemnly
by Anton Bruckner (1824–1896)

11

This is one of the longest pieces I've suggested this year, lasting around twenty-four minutes, but it's a work of such metaphysical magnitude, such transcendental scope, such preposterous humanity and such grace that if you can eke out the time, on this day or another, to give yourself over to the music completely, I would *urge* you to do so.

Main theme from *Colette*
by Thomas Adès (b. 1971)

12

I honestly can't remember the last time I heard a soundtrack before I saw the movie from which it came and decided *on the strength of the music alone* that I simply had to see the film. A longtime fan of the extraordinary British composer Thomas Adès, I'd been playing this track practically on repeat before I finally got around to seeing the film in question, *Colette*.

13

Haven
by Bryce Dessner (b.1976)

In his music, Bryce Dessner – who is better known as a member of American rock band The National – appears omnivorously sonically curious, drawing on influences from the Baroque era, folk music, Romanticism and modernist aesthetics, especially minimalism, as is evident in this enthralling and mesmeric track.

14

'Das Agnus Dei'
from *8 Sacred Songs*, op. 138
by Max Reger (1873–1916)

At not even two minutes long, this music somehow has the power to reset the world in its simplicity and beauty. The last few seconds, for example, are among the loveliest I've ever heard. I hope wherever you are you can turn up the volume and simply relish them.

Are there any lyrics or quotations that have stayed with you throughout your life? Why do you think they have resonated with you?

15

Love bade me welcome
by Judith Weir (b. 1954)

The position of Master of the Queen or King's Music has existed since 1625, when Charles I appointed a Huguenot court musician called Nicholas Lanier as head of the private band. It only took 388 years for a woman to be appointed to the post, but she got there in the end. Judith Weir writes music of intelligence and wit: she's unpretentious, full of integrity and deeply thoughtful about music's place in the world.

16

Sonata in D major
7: Passacaille
by Sylvius Leopold Weiss (1686–1750)

Sylvius Weiss was a direct contemporary of J. S. Bach, who admired his music so much he even arranged some of it. He died on this day, so it seems a fitting moment to celebrate his legacy with this beautiful and mellifluous take on the ultra-fashionable dance form of the day, the *passacaglia*.

Adagio in C minor
by Nicholas Britell (b. 1980)

17

Happy birthday to Nicholas Britell, one of the most gifted and brilliant minds on the musical scene today. This brief but devastating interlude from the hit HBO TV series *Succession* gives me shivers every time I hear it.

Liturgy of St John Chrysostom
13: 'Tebe poyem' – 'We hymn thee'
by Sergei Rachmaninov (1873–1943)

18

This is *such* radiant writing for an unaccompanied choir. Rachmaninov was a man of profound but private faith, and had apparently been contemplating setting this liturgy – which is the primary worship service of the Eastern Orthodox church – for years before he embarked upon it in 1910. Unlike with many of his compositions, divine inspiration seemed to flow from the outset.

19

Symphony no. 2 in C major, op. 61
3: Adagio espressivo
by Robert Schumann (1810–1856)

Emerging out of the silence, shrouded in mystery, laying a path for an oboe solo of breathtaking beauty and wistfulness, the opening music of this movement is one of the most gut-wrenching moments in any symphonic writing ever. It breaks my heart, every time, but in that simultaneously putting-you-back-together and redemptive way that only the very greatest music can.

20

Homages
1: 'Contemplation'
by Cheryl Frances-Hoad (b. 1980)

Time to meet another of the wonderfully distinctive voices currently lighting up contemporary British classical music – see also e.g. Charlotte Bray (10 February) and Anna Meredith (23 March). Essex-born Cheryl Frances-Hoad has been composing since she was fifteen and draws from a wide array of inspirations, including literature, poetry, painting, dance and pop music.

Doodle as you listen to the next piece of music in the book. Don't be afraid to express yourself – it's for your eyes only! – but approach it with curiosity and try to see the value of what you have created.

21

Songs of the Auvergne
2: 'Baïlèro' – 'The Shepherd's Song'
by Joseph Canteloube (1879–1957)

If you can find six or so minutes to yourself today, close your eyes and let yourself be transported to the Auvergne region of France, where Joseph Canteloube was born. If you can't, it still makes for a pretty idyllic soundtrack to modern life.

22

Autumn Leaves
by Craig Urquhart (b. 1963)

Bach, Mendelssohn, Debussy, Chopin, Schumann . . . they've all played their part when it comes to inspiring and influencing Craig Urquhart, who worked for many years as one of Leonard Bernstein's most closely trusted personal assistants and is now a composer in his own right. This piece, an ode to the season for solo piano, renders pure and sincere emotion.

Canon and Gigue in D major
1: Canon
by Johann Pachelbel (1653–1706)

23

Truth be told, I deliberated hard over whether to include this or not: it's one of the best known pieces in all classical music. You certainly don't need me to bring it back into your life. Or do you? Listen again. It's actually so, so brilliant: a complex, circular conversation between three violins, a cello, and eight bars of music repeated twenty-eight times. And how's about that *bass-line?* So good it's been pilfered by musicians through the centuries ever since. Definitely worthy of another hearing, I hope you agree.

An English Day-Book
9: 'Evening Song'
by Elizabeth Poston (1905–1987)

24

A friend to many of the leading cultural and literary lights of her time, Elizabeth Poston, who was born on this day, was a respected academic, writer and pianist as well as a fine composer. This piece comes from her *English Day-Book*, a sort of musical diary or journal in which she links together both sacred and secular poetry. The result is something quite unique.

25

Concerto Grosso in D Major, op. 6 no. 4
3: Adagio
by Arcangelo Corelli (1653–1713)

Arcangelo Corelli never lived to see published the set of concerti grossi from which this two-minute sliver of thoughtful and uplifting music comes, but every piece in the collection is an outright gem, a veritable grab bag of delights. I often stick on the entire album of Corelli's opus 6 if I need to focus, and invariably find it a deeply clarifying and fortifying listen.

26

The Seasons
Part 4: 'Autumn', no. 15: Petit Adagio
by Alexander Glazunov (1865–1936)

Such writing stills my restless heart. And such music, too: nothing quite evokes the exquisite poignancy of this time of year for me like this piece by Glazunov. Before long, at least in the northern hemisphere where I live, it will be winter: we must relish the dying embers of beautiful autumn while she lasts . . .

Which season do you most prefer, and where, and why?
Jot down the things you most enjoy/treasure in that season,
and, without expectation, think about what you might
look forward to if you get to experience it again.

27

Heartbreaker
by Missy Mazzoli (b. 1980)

Happy birthday to the American composer Missy Mazzoli, who hails from that thrilling generation who are really shaking the tree when it comes to classical music in our time. In 2018, the Grammy-nominated Mazzoli became one of the first women ever to receive a commission from New York's Metropolitan Opera.

28

Sonata in A major, Kk 208
by Domenico Scarlatti (1685–1757)

I'm an amazingly mediocre pianist, but even I can just about pick my way through this one – and I always find it an immensely meditative and nourishing experience when I do. It's four little minutes or so of clean, clarifying, music: balm for a frazzled mind and soul. I highly recommend you just stick it on wherever you are and let it do its lovely thing.

Someone to Watch Over Me
by George Gershwin (1898–1937)
arr. Joseph Turrin (b. 1947)

29

This piece, originally written for the Broadway musical *Oh, Kay!*, was first recorded on this day in 1926. I love it with all my heart – especially in this version, arranged so lusciously by the contemporary American classical composer, Joseph Turrin.

Violin Sonata no. 1 in D minor
4: Presto
by Elisabeth-Claude Jacquet de la Guerre (1665–1729)

30

Today, we meet Elizabeth-Claude Jacquet de la Guerre, who has the distinction of being the first ever Frenchwoman to produce an opera. Perhaps, it's not surprising that Jacquet de la Guerre, despite the challenges faced by any woman trying to make a name for herself in classical music, would go on to achieve great things: she was a prodigy and made her debut at the court of King Louis XIV when she was still a child.

31

From *All-Night Vigil*, op. 37
6: 'Bogoroditse Devo – Rejoice, O Virgin'
by Sergei Rachmaninov (1873–1943)

Today is All Hallows' Eve, a holiday incorporated into the Christian tradition by Pope Gregory IV in the ninth century as the eve of the Feast of All Saints. The name, which derives from the Old English 'hallowed', meaning holy or sanctified, is what gives us, of course, 'Hallowe'en'. I have resisted the urge to play spooky classical music today and have instead opted for a spine-tinglingly beautiful moment from a timeless all-night. You're welcome.

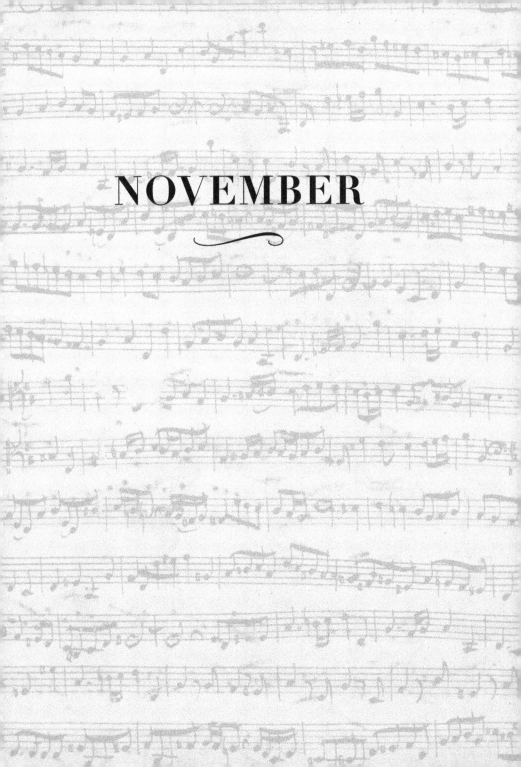

NOVEMBER

Symphony no. 9 in D minor ('Choral'), op. 125
4: Presto
by Ludwig van Beethoven (1770–1827)

1

It was on this day in 1993 that the Maastricht Treaty came into effect, marking the founding of the European Union (EU). A fitting day, then, to hear the iconic music on which the EU's official anthem is based.

Parce mihi Domine
by Cristóbal de Morales (c. 1500–1553)

2

Hugely prolific, well travelled and famous in his day, the music of Cristóbal de Morales was considered by certain critics of the time to be among the most perfect ever created. This pacifying, purifying choral work sets text from Job. It comes from Morales *Officium defunctorum* (the Office of the Dead): a prayer cycle said for the repose of the soul on All Souls' Day, which is today.

3

Notturno
by Blagoje Bersa (1873–1934)

Today we'll hear music by a largely forgotten Croatian composer who is sometimes credited with writing the first ever Croatian opera, a piece called *Oganj* from 1911. Set in a factory, it is now rarely performed but in its time it was a significant work in the post-Wagnerian mould.

Opera aside, it's Bersa's beautiful music for piano that really took my breath away. This charming and serene piece, very much in the style of the Romantic nocturne as exemplified by Chopin, is, I think, a particular neglected gem.

4

Piano Concerto in A minor, op. 16
2: Adagio
by Edvard Grieg (1843–1907)

It was whilst on holiday away from his native Norway that a twenty-four-year-old Edvard Grieg composed his magnificent piano concerto. The concerto, whose first moment has one of the most famous openings in all of music, is characterized by a tremendous vitality throughout; this bittersweet but emotionally lustrous second movement seems to overflow with feeling.

Music for the Royal Fireworks, HWV 351
4: 'La Réjouissance': Allegro
by George Frideric Handel (1685–1759)

5

Handel's *Music for the Royal Fireworks* has nothing to do with today's tradition of Guy Fawkes' Night and bonfires in Britain, but as pyrotechnical music goes, it's hard to beat. The piece was actually written to accompany a huge fireworks display in London's Green Park in 1749 to celebrate the end of the War of the Austrian Succession and the signing of the Treaty of Aix-la-Chapelle, seen as a major success for Britain at that time.

When David heard
by Thomas Tomkins (1572–1656)

6

Born in Pembrokeshire, Wales, Thomas Tomkins became one of the last members of the so-called English Virginalist school, a late Tudor/early Jacobean movement. This anguished choral work, which describes King David stricken with grief at the death of his son Absalom, was probably composed as a lament for Henry, the young Prince of Wales, who died on this day in 1612.

*Consider times you have been overly self-critical. How could you be
a little kinder to yourself? (Baby steps . . .)*

Sonata for solo harp
1: Allegretto
by Germaine Tailleferre (1892–1983)

7

When Germaine Tailleferre died, aged ninety-one, on this day, most of her music remained unpublished. That's despite the fact that she had been a prolific and dynamic figure in twentieth-century French music.

Tailleferre composed for instruments that are far less well represented in the solo canon, including saxophone, guitar, and – as in today's graceful, languid sonata from 1953 – the harp.

All Shall Be Well
by Roxanna Panufnik (b. 1968)

8

This uplifting choral work was commissioned by Bristol-based vocal ensemble the Exultate Singers for a concert celebrating twenty years since the fall of the Berlin Wall. It was first performed on this day in 2009 at Clifton Cathedral.

Panufnik weaves powerful emotion through simple, elegant harmonies – in a piece that not only makes us think, but feel. Or not only makes us feel, but think . . .

9

Cello Suite no. 2 in D minor, BWV 1008
4: Sarabande
by Johann Sebastian Bach (1685–1750)

On this morning in 1989, the celebrated cellist Mstislav Rostropovich was at home with his family in Paris when he heard reports of the Berlin Wall coming down. With all commercial flights to Berlin booked, Rostropovich called a friend with a private plane. They arrived at Checkpoint Charlie the next day. A chair procured, he sat down; took out his instrument; and as crowds of East and West Berliners gathered, began to play. It became one of the iconic, enduring images from that momentous time.

10

Pieces for keyboard, Book 4, ord. 2le, no. 3
'La Couperin'
by François Couperin (1668–1733)

The clarity and surface simplicity of this work belies the technical revolutions being quietly wreaked by its brilliant composer – not least the use of a pianist's thumbs. Seriously: before Couperin, players used only eight fingers, which seems mad to us now, but there you go!

Elegy – In memoriam Rupert Brooke
by Frederick Septimus Kelly (1881–1916)

11

In 1915 the Irish–Australian composer and Olympic rower Frederick Septimus Kelly survived the slaughter at Gallipoli, only to be killed in action at the end of the Battle of the Somme the following year. At Gallipoli, Kelly started to write this grief-stricken elegy for his friend, the poet Rupert Brooke, who had died from sepsis. Kelly was one of the group that helped bury Brooke on the Greek island of Skyros. The emotion that seeps from this restrained but aching elegy about Brooke's grave is deeply felt, then, and intensely personal.

Three pieces for two violins and piano
1: Praeludium
by Dmitri Shostakovich (1906–1975)

12

Sometimes, we all need a couple of minutes of music like this in our lives. They are among the first duets I ever played as a kid and I've loved them with all my heart ever since.

Choose a piece from the book and listen to it with your eyes closed. What do you visualize? Is it somewhere in nature, a person, an experience? Reflect on why this might be.

Ceffylau – Horses
by Catrin Finch (b. 1980) & Seckou Keita (b. 1978)

13

I was positively *thunderstruck* when I first heard the unique partnership between celebrated Welsh harpist Catrin Finch and Senegalese *kora* virtuoso Seckou Keita. Combine the harp with a kora, the traditional West African twenty-two-stringed instrument, and bam: a kind of enchantment happens! An effusive joy!

Fantasia in G minor
by Fanny Mendelssohn (1805–1847)

14

Perhaps it's because it's November, but I seem to be drawn inexorably to minor keys this month; bear with me though, because while Fanny Mendelssohn opens her *Fantasia* for cello and piano with a somewhat melancholic and brooding tonal palette, she soon ups both mood and tempo, throwing open the shades to let in light and lyricism in abundance.

15

Arcadiana, op. 12
6: 'O Albion'
by Thomas Adès (b. 1971)

To me, 'O Albion' somehow feels like an extended musical sigh, an exhalation, a reset, a rest. I return to it again and again and again; it never lets me down.

16

Sonata for harp
2: Lebhaft – Lively
by Paul Hindemith (1895–1963)

I'm reliably informed, by harpist friends, that this sonata is a joy to play. Fresh and idiomatic, it's certainly a great pleasure to listen to.

Make a list of small things that are bringing you joy throughout this month. As you start and continue this simple practice, you may see the list growing longer and longer . . .

17

Victory Stride
by James P. Johnson (1894–1955)

If you were living in America in the 1920s, the chances are you'd be familiar with a tune called 'Charleston'. It was written by James P. Johnson, who died on this day, and who invented an influential style of pianistic antics known as 'stride piano', in which the left hand leaps athletically around the keyboard. This piece is another, no less intriguing, example of Johnson's vibrant musical imagination.

18

Stars
by Ēriks Ešenvalds (b. 1977)

Choral music today from an award-winning contemporary Latvian composer. *Stars* is based on a poem by the Pulitzer Prize-winning American lyric poet Sara Teasdale (1884–1933), and the luminous simplicity and quiet intensity of her vision are, I think, matched to perfection in Ešenvalds' sublime setting. If you're wondering what the ethereal sonic glisten is throughout, it's tuned wine glasses. For real. I could listen to this forever.

Tres Romances Argentinos – Three Argentine Romances
1: 'Las niñas de Sante Fe' – 'The schoolgirls of Sante Fe'
by Carlos Guastavino (1912–2000)

Little gives me more joy than the revelation of a completely new musical discovery, and the Argentine classical composer Carlos Guastavino was a recent one of those for me. I discovered him thanks to the brilliance of Buenos Aires-born pianist Martha Argerich, whose performance of this gorgeous, sensual and unashamedly romantic dance is an absolute gift.

Part 3: 'Invisible Light: Earth Seen from Above' from *Atlas*
by Meredith Monk (b.1942)

20

This ethereal track, composed in 1987, is a rapturous seven or so minutes, elevating us, as the title promises, to another plane – one of sublime perspective.

21

momentary (choir version)
by Ólafur Arnalds (b. 1986)

From my heart to yours: this shimmering choral fragment; and the sheer marvellous miracle, frankly, of this, of this just being here, momentarily.

I have no further words.

22

Evensong
by Liza Lehmann (1862–1918)

Let us raise a toast, today, to the first president of the Society of Women Musicians and an indomitable force in the music of her time, much admired by the great Clara Schumann, although these days she is inevitably mostly dismissed by classical purists as a mere composer of 'light' music.

Note down the composers that have most inspired you with both their music and their story. What are the qualities they express? What is it about these people that you feel is so inspirational?

23

Spem in alium – 'Hope in another'
by Thomas Tallis (1505–1585)

A ten-minute unaccompanied choral work in which Tallis inter-twines forty separate voices in a tapestry of supreme complexity yet absolute radiance. *Spem in alium* is often held up as a sort of vision-ary pinnacle of the genre, and rightly so.

24

Magnetic Rag – *Synchopations Classiques*
by Scott Joplin (c. 1868–1917)

It twists my heart a little, to think that this was the last rag that Scott Joplin would ever write. By the time he produced it he was already ravaged by the latter stages of syphilis that would kill him three years later. It has a dark, melancholic middle section and yet, because it's Joplin, and because he was a genius, it's also infectiously wonderful, full of sincerest feeling and joy.

Adagio for Strings
by Samuel Barber (1910–1981)

25

The *Adagio*, adapted from the slow movement of Samuel Barber's 1936 string quartet, was used at the funerals of Albert Einstein, Princess Grace, and at official memorials for Diana, Princess of Wales and the victims of the 9/11 terrorist attacks.

The piece has become shorthand for unutterable sorrow. I'll let the music speak for itself.

Music for Pieces of Wood
by Steve Reich (b. 1936)

26

A terrific example, today, of music that does what it says on the tin: this indeed is music for pieces of wood, no more, no less. Each player has a pair of wooden claves, the sorts of cylindrical pieces of hard wood you might find in a toddler's toy box, here selected for their particular pitches and resonant timbre. I'll never forget the first time I ever heard this: it has lost none of its capacity to thrill.

27

L'amante segreto – The Secret Lover
'Voglio, voglio morire' – 'I want to die'
by Barbara Strozzi (1619–1677)

There's not a huge amount of biographical information to be found about the prolific Venetian singer, composer and poet Barbara Strozzi. In the two decades between 1644 and 1664, we know that she published hundreds of songs: this 1651 song nails a situation that I suspect many of us have probably been through (as teenagers, if not since!). Namely: when you're in love with the wrong person, and would frankly rather *die* than have the object of your affection ever find out how you feel . . . Yup. You too?

28

Some
by Nils Frahm (b. 1982)

I often find myself sending Frahm tracks to friends and loved ones and colleagues, or even just to people I meet who ask me for a certain piece of music to match a certain need or manage a certain mood. There is something not only incredibly sonically diverse about his music, but emotive and empathic too. In other words, it connects.

Think about a time when you've been in love, or perhaps when you first fell in love. This is an enormous question, obviously: but what does love mean to you? Even asking the question might help clarify your innermost feelings and priorities.

29

Eve
by Amelia Warner (b. 1982)

The atmospheric track I've chosen for this late-November day comes from Amelia Warner's 2017 EP *Visitors*, each track of which is based on a fictional female character. She plays piano and organ on the record, which is also scored for violin, viola, cello and double bass.

30

Maria Magdalena
by Francisco Guerrero (1528–1599)

When wintry nights are drawing in, I find there's nothing like a spot of sublime Renaissance polyphony to warm the soul and for me, today's composer invariably hits the spot.

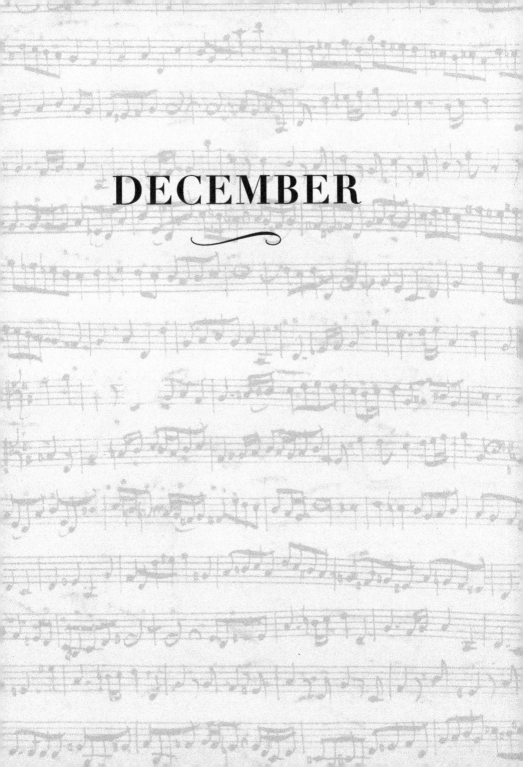

DECEMBER

O Magnum Mysterium
by Morten Lauridsen (b. 1943)

Well, hello December. The last month of our musical year. To set the tone for the festive season, I wanted to start with one of the most beautiful nativity settings I have ever heard . . .

In Paradisum
by Galina Grigorjeva (b. 1962)

I particularly love this treatment by the Ukraine-born Estonian composer Galina Grigorjeva, whose birthday it is today. The In Paradisum is a part of the Latin Western liturgical Requiem Mass. So it's inevitably religiously inflected, yes, but in her hands never dogmatic: full of subtle sonorities and richness, deeply felt yet somehow light of touch.

3

Sonata for violin and continuo
3: *Imitazione delle campane*
by Johann Paul von Westhoff (1656–1705)
arr. Christian Badzura (b. 1977)

For my money, this piece is one of the most stunning works to emerge from the Baroque era. With its eerie opening, hypnotic bassline and crunchy dissonances, this movement stopped me in my tracks when I first encountered it, and no matter how many times I hear it, I am never not mesmerized. I find myself returning to it again and again.

4

Come, Holy Ghost
by Jonathan Harvey (1939–2012)

Today's music, a beautiful hymn written by the British composer Jonathan Harvey in 1984, is a timeless distillation of the mystery that animates all life. This is also unabashedly 'modern music', whatever that means.

Music for Strings
2: 'The Last Words of M'
by Isobel Waller-Bridge (b. 1984)

5

Waller-Bridge, an award-winning young British composer, writes beautifully crafted and narratively potent music, often for film and television (including her sister Phoebe's now-iconic series *Fleabag*).

Today she is very much tapping into the British tradition of writing expansive, filmic, emotionally searing music for strings – which is, as it happens, the name of the splendid 2015 album from which this track comes.

8 pieces for clarinet, viola and piano, op. 83
6: 'Nachtgesang': Andante con moto
by Max Bruch (1838–1920)

6

Bruch wrote his first piece aged eleven, and by fourteen had completed a symphony and a prize-winning string quartet. He went on to have a major career as a conductor, composer and pedagogue. The suite of pieces from which this profoundly expressive nocturne comes was written in 1909 as a gift for his son Max Felix. I find the combination of instruments deliciously sensuous and mellow, and the pleasure I take in listening to it is only deepened by the tender thought that it was created by a father, lovingly, for a son.

Many people around the world will be celebrating Advent now. How does your family celebrate the holidays? Think about any cherished personal traditions. Are there new ones you hope to introduce in the future? Or ones that remind you of loved ones who are no longer here?

In the Mists
1: Andante
by Leoš Janáček (1854–1928)

7

Leoš Janáček didn't write a lot of piano music, but what he did is wonderfully distinctive. Rather than peddling the sort of technical pyrotechnics many composers feel compelled to conjure on a keyboard, he instead goes for maximum atmosphere. I love the brooding, evocative opening of his last work for piano, the cycle *In the Mists*, whose first public performance took place on this day in 1913.

From *Sleep*
'Dream 3 (in the midst of my life)'
by Max Richter (b. 1966)

8

I wish I could find a way to explain what happened when I first experienced Richter's extraordinary music live, but it's impossible. Words elude me. The best I can say is that I seemed to transcend my standard plane of existence and was transported into another dimension. It felt like ecstasy. It felt like a miracle. It felt like everything.

9

Oboe Concerto in B flat major, Wq. 164
1: Allegretto
by Carol Philip Emanuel Bach (1714–1788)

The fifth child and second surviving son of Johann Sebastian Bach, 'C. P. E.', as he tends to be known, was once more famous and more revered even than his genius of a father.

His lyrical, melodic and expressive music made him a leading exponent of what became known as the 'sensitive style'. I love that.

10

Prelude, Fugue and Variation in B minor, FWV 30, op. 18
1. Prelude – Andantino cantabile
by César Franck (1822–1890)
transcribed for piano by Harold Bauer (1873–1951)

If the biographies and contemporary character reports are to be believed, Franck was a particularly kindhearted soul. His great friend, the fellow composer Camille Saint-Saëns, was the dedicatee of today's piece. I love its gentle opening movement, especially as transcribed for the piano: its tinges of melancholy, and its pathos.

Piano Concerto no. 18 in B flat major, K. 456
1: Allegro vivace
by Wolfgang Amadeus Mozart (1756–1791)

11

Selecting a Mozart piano concerto was a sort of torment. How, how to choose?

In the end I could not in good faith recommend one over another, so I've cheated and gone for the concerto Mozart likely wrote for Maria-Theresia von Paradis. Please consider this a diving-off point and explore them all!

Jesus Christ the Apple Tree
by Elizabeth Poston (1905–1987)

12

With under a fortnight to go until Christmas, we can surely permit ourselves a little carol?

Mid December is a time to rest and build strength for the challenges of the coming year. Use mindfulness to help you prioritize the taking of a little time for yourself. Plan five acts of meaningful self care to undertake over the next few months.

Concerto Grosso in G minor ('Christmas Concerto'), op. 6 no. 8
2: Adagio – Allegro – Adagio
by Arcangelo Corelli (1653–1713)

13

Sticking with the festive mood, I thought today would be a good day to hear a piece by Arcangelo Corelli known as the 'Christmas Concerto' because its manuscript bears the inscription *'Fatto per la notte di Natale'* – 'Made for the night of Christmas'.

Consider it an early Christmas gift.

Upon Your Heart
by Eleanor Daley (b. 1955)

14

Sometimes, the best things in life are just simple truths. Not that Canadian composer Eleanor Daley's beautiful choral composition is in any way *simplistic*.

There is something so incredibly restorative and quietly comforting in the sound of unadorned human voices singing together; the way it re-establishes a connection with a part of your inner landscape. I think this is a perfect example.

15

Lágrima
by Francisco Tárrega (1852–1909)

Sometimes music falls into your life in the most serendipitous and unlikely of ways. It was on a miserable tube journey at rush hour in London that I first encountered this piece, which has gone on to be one of my favourite works for classical guitar.

16

Noël
by Augusta Holmès (1847–1903)

It was on this day that the composer of this particular festive song, Augusta Holmès, was born, to Irish parents, in Paris. In her early career, like so many female artists, Holmès struggled to be taken seriously. (Rumour has it that the composer's mother expressly forbade her passion for music, and that, despairing, the young Augusta tried to kill herself.) Either way, we do know that she chose to employ the pseudonym 'Hermann Zenta' for her earliest compositions, presumably for its Mitteleuropean air of 'seriousness'.

The Three Kings
by Jonathan Dove (b. 1959)

17

A setting of a seasonal poem written in 1916 by the fascinating English crime novelist – oh, and short-story writer, playwright, essayist, linguist, translator of Dante, good friend of C. S. Lewis, early advertising maven, and so on – Dorothy L. Sayers, who died on this day in 1957.

The masterly British composer Jonathan Dove brings something distinctive – haunting, layered, new – to complement the text.

Il neige – It is Snowing
by Henrique Oswald (1852–1931)

18

Maybe, depending which country, continent, or hemisphere you are reading this in, there is a chance of snow today . . . Either way, I sincerely hope you can enjoy this musical sketch of the white stuff, by a regrettably sidelined but very important Brazilian composer.

19

La Fiesta de la Posada
by Dave Brubeck (1920–2012)

Dave Brubeck was 'supposed' to be a cattle rancher, like his father. So he went to college to study veterinary science. Realizing his mind wasn't in it, his zoology professor ordered him to join the music conservatory instead. Brubeck changed course and the rest is history . . .

Brubeck was a genius. His astonishing legacy in jazz history means we rarely hear his ventures into classical, but today we have a seasonal piece of his, *The Posada*, a traditional Mexican re-enactment of Mary and Joseph's search for lodgings in Bethlehem.

20

Cradle Song
by Michael Berkeley (b. 1948)

Inching closer to Christmas, it's time for another carol: this one by the multi-talented and multi-award-winning composer, author and broadcaster Michael Berkeley. This godson of Benjamin Britten (13 June) writes opera, ballet and instrumental music, and as a former chorister, is steeped in the glories of Britain's long and illustrious choral tradition.

Try to take time during the Winter Solstice to pause and reflect. Think about what you set out to achieve this year and write this down. Is there anything you wish you had done? If so, can you add it to your list of intentions for next year? Consider how you might make it happen.

21

Outrage at Valdez
by Frank Zappa (1940–1993)

In 1989, legendary French aquatic explorer, scientist, diver and innovator Jacques Cousteau made a documentary, *Outrage at Valdez*, about the recent environmental disaster caused when an Exxon tanker hit a reef in Prince William Sound, Alaska, pouring 11 million gallons of crude oil into the sea. And the equally legendary experimental, creative artist Frank Zappa, born on this day, was tasked to provide some music for the soundtrack. The result is quite something.

22

Lachrimae
by John Dowland (1563–1626)

Today we travel to a completely different sound world, as we are transported back through the centuries to one of the most acclaimed musical figures of the Renaissance era. John Dowland was a high priest of melancholy, writing works, mostly for the lute, that tug persistently on the heartstrings. Like all the very best sad music, though, it invariably has the effect of lifting the spirits and I can't get enough of it.

'Little Serenade'
by Peter Sculthorpe (1929–2014)

23

Peter Sculthorpe stated that he wanted his music to make people feel better and happier for having listened to it. That's certainly the effect on me of this lovely little serenade, originally written in 1978 for string quartet, but orchestrated wonderfully in alternative versions.

Missa De Apostolis
Agnus Dei
by Heinrich Isaac (c. 1450/55–1517)

24

It cannot be overstated how rare it must have been to enjoy a multi-decade-long, internationally acclaimed, not to mention seriously influential career as a living composer . . . in the fifteenth century! I mean, it is pretty rare now, but imagine five-hundred-plus years ago! But that is what Heinrich Isaac managed to achieve. It must have helped that he wrote music of spine-tingling emotional power, like this.

Music is often at the heart of times of celebration. It can bring people together and can evoke memories and thoughts of loved ones who are no longer with us. Make time on this special day for yourself and the music. Close your eyes and listen. Acknowledge any feelings, whether they are joyful or sad. Memory is a powerful thing. It has the potential to heal painful aspects of our lives, restore our equilibrium and give us renewed resolve for the future.

Dormi, Jesu
by John Rutter (b. 1945)

25

John Rutter is associated with Christmas, having composed or arranged dozens of carols and other seasonal fare. For today, I have chosen one that was written in 1999 for the choir of King's College, Cambridge to perform during the college's Festival of Nine Lessons and Carols.

Siete canciones populares españolas
5: 'Nana'
by Manuel de Falla (1876–1946)

26

Our human instinct to transmit solace in a melody, to soothe through music, goes very deep; parents from all cultures have been singing lullabies to their babies for ever, often, seemingly instinctively, using the same sorts of rocking rhythms and gentle vocal inflections no matter where they come from or what age they live in.

Sometimes, with these great composers, I think we run the risk of forgetting that they are just like us – children, parents, people. An acoustic bridge indeed.

27
O Gaúcho (Corta-jaca)
by Francisca Edwiges Neves 'Chiquinha' Gonzaga
(1847–1935)

The illegitimate daughter of a mixed-race mother and white father, Chiquinha Gonzaga overcame spectacular odds to become one of Brazil's greatest musical pioneers. Defying her family and the husband she'd been forced to marry, she forged an impressive career as a pianist and composer and became her country's first ever female conductor. An ardent suffragist, she campaigned against slavery and helped to found a performers' rights collecting society. She was still writing operas in 1934, the year before she died.

28
Piano Sonata in C major, Hob. XVI no. 50
1: Allegro
by Joseph Haydn (1732–1809)

Just in case you've fallen into the post-Christmas stupor that I invariably find myself in at this time of year, this crisp and fizzy little keyboard number from Haydn should do the trick.

In the Bleak Midwinter
by Gustav Holst (1874–1934)
arr. Sheku Kanneh-Mason (b. 1999)

29

Today's piece was already a beloved wintry fixture – with its stirringly evocative words by the Pre-Raphaelite British poet Christina Rossetti, who died on this day, and music by illustrious British composer Gustav Holst. Then, in 2018, the British musician Sheku Kanneh-Mason arranged this for cello and piano. His short arrangement is spare, emotionally charged, technically breathtaking, playful, mournful. One minute you want to laugh with glee at its sheer brilliance; the next your heartstrings are being properly tugged.

The long day closes
by Arthur Sullivan (1842–1900)

30

The name Arthur Sullivan may not perhaps ring bells, but the chances are you'll have heard of Gilbert and Sullivan, a British partnership almost as iconic as the Marks and Spencer brand, or fish and chips. Before he was one half of that legendary operetta-producing machine, Sullivan was a talented and prolific composer of 'part-songs' – written for several vocal parts – which were all the rage in Victorian England. I find this one, with its plaintive harmonies and touching sentiment, particularly lovely.

31

Trumpet Voluntary, op. 6 no. 5
by John Stanley (1712–1786)

Whatever your New Year's Eve celebrations look like this year, or any year hence: I am here to remind you that you are . . . alive. You made it. And that alone is cause for celebration.

This may sound like a platitude, but I *really mean it*. No matter how privileged or fortunate you might be compared to some other people, life is hard. So deep breath. Raise your glass. Humans are incredible.

Happy new year.

Try to take stock of your listening year. What a time we've had! Go back to page 20 and remind yourself how you felt back in January. I sincerely hope you notice a sense of growth and accomplishment. Thank you for accompanying me on our musical trip around the sun, and I wish you all the best with the next chapter of your life's journey. See you next year?

Index

265